CURRENT CONCEPTS IN REGIONAL ANAESTHESIA

DEVELOPMENTS IN CRITICAL CARE MEDICINE AND ANESTHESIOLOGY

Prakash, O. (ed.): Applied Physiology in Clinical Respiratory Care. 1982. ISBN 90-247-2662-X.

McGeown, Mary G.: Clinical Management of Electrolyte Disorders. 1983. ISBN 0-89838-559-8.

Scheck, P.A., Sjöstrand, U.H., and Smith, R.B. (eds.): Perspectives in High Frequency Ventilation. 1983. ISBN 0-89838-571-7.

Stanley, T.H., and Petty, W.C. (eds.): New Anesthetic Agents, Devices and Monitoring Techniques. 1983. ISBN 0-89838-566-0.

Prakash, O. (ed.): Computing in Anesthesia and Intensive Care. 1983. ISBN 0-89838-602-0.

Stanley, T.H., and Petty, W.C. (eds.): Anesthesia and the Cardiovascular System. 1984. ISBN 0-89838-626-8.

Van Kleef, J.W., Burm, A.G.L., and Spierdijk, J. (eds.): Current Concepts in Regional Anaesthesia. 1984. ISBN 0-89838-644-6.

CURRENT CONCEPTS IN REGIONAL ANAESTHESIA

Proceedings of the second general meeting of the European Society of Regional Anaesthesia

edited by

JACK W. VAN KLEEF, MD
ANTON G.L. BURM, MSc
JOHAN SPIERDIJK, MD

Department of Anaesthesiology
Leiden University Hospital
Leiden, The Netherlands

1984 **MARTINUS NIJHOFF PUBLISHERS**
a member of the KLUWER ACADEMIC PUBLISHERS GROUP
BOSTON / THE HAGUE / DORDRECHT / LANCASTER
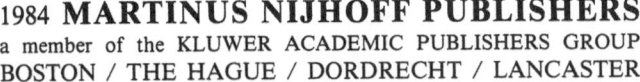

Distributors

for the United States and Canada: Kluwer Boston, Inc., 190 Old Derby Street, Hingham, MA 02043, USA
for all other countries: Kluwer Academic Publishers Group, Distribution Center, P.O.Box 322, 3300 AH Dordrecht, The Netherlands

Library of Congress Cataloging in Publication Data

European Society of Regional Anaesthesia. General
    Meeting (2nd : 1983 : Leiden, Netherlands)
    Current concepts in regional anaesthesia.

    (Developments in critical care medicine and anaes-
thesiology)
    Includes index.
    1. Conduction anesthesia--Congresses. I. Kleef,
Jack W. van. II. Burm, Anton G. L. III. Spierdijk, Joh.
IV. Title. V. Series.
RD84.E88 1983   617'.964   84-4108

ISBN-13: 978-94-009-6017-6   e-ISBN-13: 978-94-009-6015-2
DOI: 10.1007/978-94-009-6015-2

Copyright

PREFACE

This book contains the papers that were presented at the 2nd
general meeting of the European Society of Regional Anaesthesia
(E.S.R.A.) which was held in Leiden on September 1st, 2nd and
3rd 1983. During the meeting a fruitful exchange of knowledge
was initiated which I hope will lead to further inspiration
and research. The book covers the following topics:
- Special Blocks
- Obstetric Pathology
- Epidural versus Spinal Anaesthesia
- (Postoperative) Pain Control
I would like to express my gratitude to all the speakers who sent
their manuscripts in time for publishing. I should also like to
thank the co-editors of this book, as well as mr B.F. Commandeur,
from Martinus Nijhoff Publishers for their cooperation. Finally
I should like to express my gratitude especially to Mrs J.I.
Tieleman-Shamir for all her secretarial work, and to Miss
M.P.M. Toelen for typing a good number of the manuscripts.

Jack W. van Kleef

CONTENTS

VIII

FACULTY

Prof. P.R. Bromage
Department of Anesthesiology
University of Colorado
Health Sciences Center
4200 East Ninth Avenue
Denver/Colorado 80262
U.S.A.

A.G.L. Burm M.Sc.
Afdeling Anaesthesiologie
Academisch Ziekenhuis
Rijnsburgerweg 10
2333 AA Leiden/The Netherlands

Prof. H.U. Gerbershagen
Schmerz Zentrum Mainz
Alice Hospital
Auf der Steig 14-16
6500 Mainz 1/West Germany

Prof. N.M. Greene
Department of Anesthesiology
Yale University/School of Medicine
Yale New Haven Hospital
333 Cedar Street
New Haven/Connecticut 06510
U.S.A.

Dr. J.G. Hannington-Kiff
Pain Relief Clinic
Frimley Park Hospital
Portsmouth Road
Frimley/Surrey GU16 5UJ
United Kingdom

Prof.A.I. Hollmen
Department of Anaesthesiology
University of Oulu
90100 Oulu 10/Finland

Mrs. Dr. J.P. Holm
Kliniek voor obstetrie en gynaecologie
Academisch Ziekenhuis
Oostersingel 59
9713 EZ Groningen/The Netherlands

Dr. R.H.W.M. van den Hoogen
Afdeling Anaesthesiologie
Diaconessenhuis
Houtlaan 55
2334 CK Leiden

Dr. H. Kehlet
Kommunehospitalet
Surgical Department 1
Østen Farimagsgade 5
1399 Copenhagen K/Denmark

Prof. M.J.N.C. Keirse
Vrouwenkliniek
Academisch Ziekenhuis
Rijnsburgerweg 10
2333 AA Leiden/The Netherlands

Dr. J.W. van Kleef
Afdeling Anaesthesiologie
Academisch Ziekenhuis
Rijnsburgerweg 10
2333 AA Leiden/The Netherlands

Dr. J.T.A. Knape
Gansoord 4
1411 RH Naarden/The Netherlands

Dr. E. Lanz
Institut für Anaesthesiologie
der Universität
6500 Mainz/West Germany

Dr. D.C. Moore
Department of Anesthesiology
The Mason Clinic
118 Ninth Avenue
Seattle/Washington 98101
U.S.A.

Prof. H. Nolte
Institut für Anaesthesiologie
Klinikum Minden
Bismarckstrasse 6 - Bereich 1
4950 Minden/Westfalen
West Germany

Prof. H. Renck
Department of Anaesthesia
Malmö Allmänna Sjukhus
21401 Malmö/Sweden

Dr. O. Schulte-Steinberg
Dietrichweide 7
D-8135 Söcking/West Germany

Dr. D.B. Scott
Department of Anaesthetics
Royal Infirmary of Edinburgh
Lauriston Place
Edinburgh EH3 9YW/United Kingdom

Dr. S.J. Seddon
Department of Anaesthetics
City General Hospital
New Castle Road
Stoke on Trent ST4 6QG
United Kingdom

Prof. Joh. Spierdijk
Afdeling Anaesthesiologie
Academisch Ziekenhuis
Rijnsburgerweg 10
2333 AA Leiden/The Netherlands

Prof. M. D'A. Stanton-Hicks
Institut für Anaesthesiologie
Medizinische Einrichtungen der
Universität Düsseldorf
Moorenstrasse 5
4000 Düsseldorf 1/West Germany

Dr. A. van Steenberge
Vliertjeslaan 11
1900 Overijse/Belgium

Prof. P. Stieglitz
Departement d'Anesthesie Reanimation
Centre Hospitalier Regional et
Universitaire de Grenoble
38043 Grenoble Cedex/France

Dr. G.T. Tucker
Department of Therapeutics
Hallamshire Hospital
Glossop Road
Sheffield S10 2JF/United Kingdom

Prof. J.B. Weiss
Brigham and Women's Hospital
Department of Obstetric Anesthesia
75 Francis Street
Boston/Massachusetts 02115
U.S.A.

Dr. L. Wiklund
Department of Anesthesiology
University Hospital
S 751 85 Uppsala/Sweden

MULTIPLE INTERCOSTAL BLOCKS BY A SINGLE INJECTION? - A CLINICAL AND RADIOLOGICAL INVESTIGATION

H. RENCK, A. JOHANSSON, P. ASPELIN, AND H. JACOBSEN

INTRODUCTION

Intercostal nerve blocks have since long been a routine procedure in our institution. Like many others[1-12] we have found these blocks to provide a very effective pain relief in various clinical situations causing few side effects[13-18].

However, when these blocks are performed with the conventional technique they carry the disadvantages of multiple and painful injections at a site which requires turning of the patients. This makes prolongation by repetitive blocks cumbersome to the patients as well as to the personell.

It was therefore with great interest we noticed the report by Nunn and Slavin[19] which described the anatomy of the inter-costal space. The authors stated that an intercostal injection spreads medially into the paravertebral space and is free to pass over the internal aspect of the rib to the adjacent inter-costal spaces. Prolonged blockade of multiple intercostal nerves would thus be possible by repetitive or continuous administration of local anaesthetics through a single catheter inserted into one intercostal space.

The aim of the present study was to investigate the anatomical spread of a large volume of a local anaesthetic injected into one intercostal space as well as the distribution of the resulting cutaneous analgesia.

MATERIAL AND METHODS

Five volunteering anaesthesiologists underwent percutaneous catheterisation of the 9th intercostal space on one side and of the subcostal space on the other. The procedure was performed

2

at the costal angle employing a Touhy needle and an epidural
catheter. The catheters were injected with a mixture of 16 ml
0.25% Marcaine with adrenaline, 5 ug/ml, and 4 ml of a contrast
medium (Hexabrix[R]). The anatomical spread of the injection
was evaluated by computer tomography (CT).

On separate occasions the volunteers also underwent separate
blocks of the 7th to 11th intercostal nerves using a total
volume of 20 ml 0.5% Marcaine with adrenaline, 5 ug/ml, and
an injection of 20 ml of the local anaesthetic into the 9th
intercostal space. All injections took place at the costal
angle. The distribution of cutaneous analgesia and hypalgesia
was evaluated by pin prick at regular intervals.

RESULTS

The typical spread of an injection of 20 ml into the 9th
intercostal space can be seen in fig 1-4. At vertebral levels
T8 and T9 the mixture is located posterior to the ribs. At the
T10 level a "flattening" of the parietal pleura is shown
indicating an expansion of the 9th intercostal space. At the
T11 level the mixture is located posterior to the intercostal
space.

The result of an injection into the subcostal space is seen
in fig 5-9. At vertebral level T12-L1 essentially no contrast
can be seen on the left side - the contrast on the right side
emanates from the injection into the 9th intercostal space on
that side. At vertebral levels L2 and L3 the contrast is
located within the quadratus lumborum muscle and at the L4
level no contrast can be seen.

In no case could any spread of the injection be seen to
either the paravertebral space or from one intercostal space
to another.

After separate blocks of intercostal nerves 7 to 11 cutaneous
hypalgesia or analgesia occurred according to fig 9. The latency
to regression to three segments was 4.0 ± 2.0 hours and to one
segment 6.8 ± 2.8 hours. Only a few segments were blocked
following injection of 20 ml of the local anaesthetic into the
9th intercostal space (fig 10). Only the latency to regression
to one segment could be calculated, 7.2 ± 4.3 hours, which is

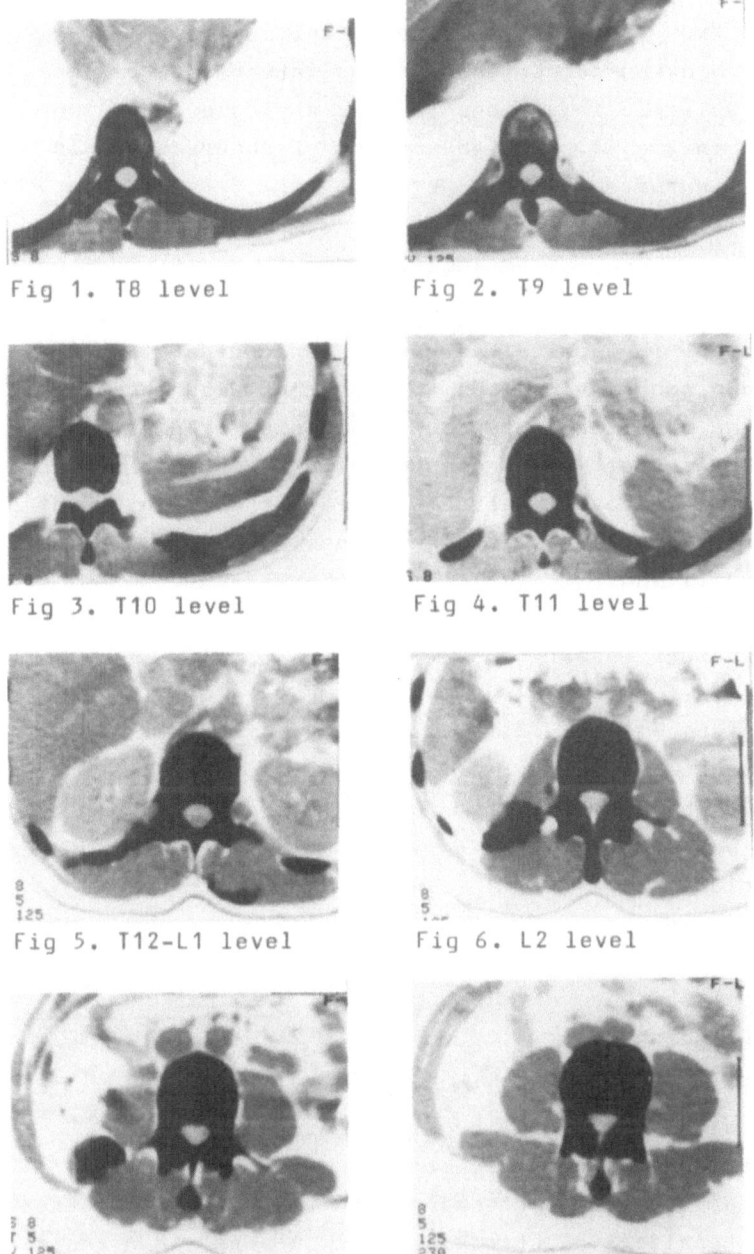

Fig 1. T8 level

Fig 2. T9 level

Fig 3. T10 level

Fig 4. T11 level

Fig 5. T12-L1 level

Fig 6. L2 level

Fig 7. L3 level

Fig 8. L4 level

not different from the value obtained after multiple injections.
The number of blocked segments following intercostal blocks
performed by multiple injections (—) or a single injection
(--) is given in fig 11. M$\pm$SD and number of observations is
given in the figures.

DISCUSSION

    Our finding that a large volume of a local anaesthetic
injected into one intercostal space does not spread to the
place of adjacent intercostal nerves is in contrast to the
opinion of Nunn and Slavin[19] but in agreement with the report
of Moore[20]. The resulting cutaneous analgesia is in all cases
restricted to three or less segments which - considering the
overlapping of intercostal nerves - implies that no block of
surrounding intercostal nerves takes place.

    Somewhat surprisingly
the duration of analgesia
is the same whether the
intercostal space is
injected with 20 or 4 ml
of the local anaesthetic.
This finding might indicate
that a major portion of
the larger volume is
distributed outside
the intercostal space
which also could be
seen on the CT scans.

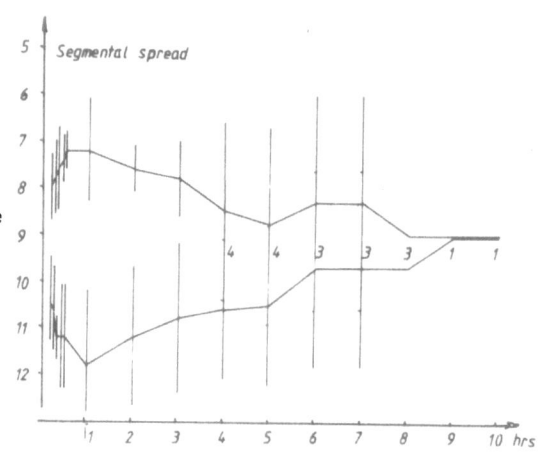

Fig 9

    From a clinical point of wiev it is our opinion that
multiple intercostal blocks result in a more satisfactory
analgesia after i e cholecystectomy than the single injection
technique. In earlier investigations[10,11] it was shown that
the majority of patients require only one set of intercostal
blocks for satisfactory pain relief during the first 20 hours
after cholecystectomy. According to Murphy[21] 92% of the
patients require no additional analgesia when intercostal
block is repeated via a single catheter inserted into the 7th

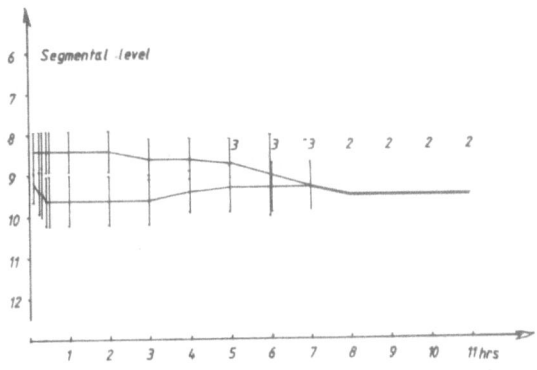

Fig 10

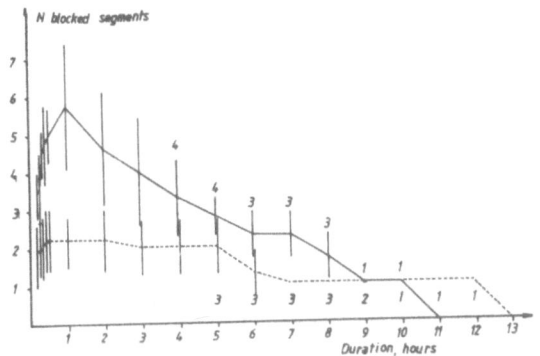

Fig 11

or 8th intercostal space. However, according to our results
a more adequate spread of cutaneous analgesia is obtained when
blocks are performed in the conventional way.

We as well as others[22,23] have found the technique to be
useful in patients with multiple fractured ribs. Whether
analgesia in these cases is accomplished by spread of the
local anaesthetic to the fracture hematoma or by its systemic
effects is not known.

In summary the singel catheter technique offers possibilities
to prolonged blockade of only a few segments. For pain relief
after cholecystectomy this might be of some value but according
to our opinion one or two sets of multiple intercostal blocks

is to be preferred.

REFERENCES

1. Moore DC, Bridenbaugh DL. 1962. Intercostal nerve block in 4333 patients: indications, technique and complications. Anesth Analg 41,1.
2. Ablondi MA, Ryan JF, O'Connell CT, Haley RW. 1966. Continuous intercostal nerve blocks for postoperative pain relief. Anesth Analg 45,185.
3. Jörgensen H. 1967. Intercostalblockad med LAC-43 (Marcain) efter cholecystectomi. Nord Med 78(41),1325.
4. Hollmén A, Saukkonen J. 1969. Zur postoperativen Schmerz-ausschaltung nach oberbauchoperationen. Narcotica, Inter-costalblockade und Epiduralanaesthesie und deren Einfluss auf die Atmung. Der Anaesthesist 18(9),298.
5. Quimby ChW. 1972. Intercostal - celiac plexus block for abdominal surgery in the poor risk patient. J Ark Med Soc 68(9),266.
6. Bridenbaugh PO, Bridenbaugh LD, Moore DC, Thompson GE. 1972. The role of intercostal block and three general anesthetic agents as predisposing factors to postoperative pulmonary problems. Anesth Analg 51(4),638.
7. Bridenbaugh PO, DuPen SL, Moore DC et al. 1973. Post-operative intercostal nerve block analgesia versus narcotic analgesia. Anesth Analg 52(1),81.
8. Engberg G. 1975. Single-shot intercostal nerve blocks with etidocaine for pain relief after upper abdominal surgery. Acta anaesth scand suppl 60,43.
9. Cronin KD, Davies MJ. 1976. Intercostal block for post-operative pain relief. Anaesth Int Care 4(3),259.
10. Renck H, Kinnberger B, Zell J-Å. 1977. Intercostal nerve block and intermittent administration of meperidine: a comparision of their effects on the early post-operative course with special reference to PEFR and VMA excretion. Opmear 22,27.
11. Andrén-Sandberg Å, Johansson BG, Renck H. 1977. Plasma cholesterol and plasma proteins in postoperative patients - a comparision between patients under conventional analgesic regime and patients receiving intermittent intercostal and splanchnic blocks. Opmear 22,151.
12. Engberg G. 1983. Intercostal block for prevention of pulmonary complications after upper abdominal surgery. Acta anaesth scand suppl 27,73.
13. Moore DC, Bridenbaugh LD. 1962. Pneumothorax. Its incidence following intercostal nerve block. JAMA 182(10),1005.
14. Benumof JL. Semenza J. 1975. Total spinal anesthesia following intrathoracic intercostal nerve blocks. Anesthesiology 43(1),124.
15. Moore DC, Mather LE, Bridenbaugh PO et al. 1976. Arterial and venous plasma levels of bupivacaine following epidural and intercostal nerve blocks. Anesthesilogy 45(1),39.

16. Jakobson S. 1977. Intercostal nerve blocks and chest wall mechanics. Abstracts of Uppsala Dissertations from the Faculty of Medicine 270.
17. Cottrell WM. 1978. Hemodynamic changes after intercostal nerve block with bupivacaine-epinephrine solution. Anesth Analg 57,492.
18. Brodsky JB. 1979. Hypotension from intraoperative intercostal nerve blocks. Reg Anesth 4,17.
19. Nunn JF, Slavin G. 1980. Posterior intercostal nerve block for pain relief after cholecystectomy. Anatomical basis and efficacy. Br J Anaesth 52,253.
20. Moore DC. 1981. Intercostal nerve block: spread of india ink injected to the ribs costal groove. Br J Anaesth 53, 325.
21. Murphy DF. 1983. Continuous intercostal nerve blockade for pain relief following cholecystectomy. Br J Anaesth 55,521.
22. O'Kelly E, Garry B. 1981. Continuous pain relief for multiple fractured ribs. Br J Anaesth 53,989.
23. Guldmann N. 1982. Continuous intercostal nerve block. Ugeskr Laeger 144,2423.

AN ALTERNATIVE METHOD OF INTERCOSTAL BLOCK
(STUDIES OF THE USE OF THE JET INJECTOR)

S.J. SEDDON

1. INTRODUCTION

Intercostal nerve block is a simple technique which can provide useful analgesia for large areas of the thoracic and abdominal wall. Although it is not so difficult to perform as some other nerve blocks it suffers two important disadvantages which have limited its wider use. Firstly, if the source of pain is extensive, multiple injections on both sides of the body may be necessary and this may discourage the inexperienced doctor, who would probably find it easier to prescribe a single injection of Morphine or similar drug.

Secondly, and perhaps more importantly, there is always a risk of causing pneumothorax. In reality this risk is slight – experts who use the technique frequently quote rates of lower than one in 1000 blocks, but nevertheless, pneumothorax is a potentially very dangerous complication and one can hardly blame doctors who are unfamiliar with the technique for being put off.

As long as a needle is used there is always a risk that the pleura will be penetrated and a pneumothorax may result. Only if the injection could be performed without using a needle would the risk of pneumothorax be avoided.

Jet injectors were originally developed for mass vaccination programmes. This is the only system available today for injecting drugs without using a needle and the studies to be described are of the use of a jet injector to perform intercostal nerve block.

2. TECHNICAL ASPECTS OF JET INJECTION

In essence, jet injectors are powerful water pistols. Fluid is driven through a very narrow orifice at a sufficient pressure to penetrate skin. The motive power can be compressed gas or a spring.

In the studies to be described the injector used was the Med-E-Jet. This gun uses a cylinder of carbon dioxide housed in its handle as the power source. When the trigger is pulled a driving piston is exposed to the pressure of gas in the cylinder. If a pressure of 100,000 KPa (300psi) is reached the piston is then released. It travels forward until its movement is arrested by a mechanical stop whose position can be varied to regulate the dose of fluid delivered. The piston is connected to a detachable and autoclavable head which contains the fluid to be injected. As the piston moves forward the fluid is forced through an orifice of 0.2 mm diameter and this fluid now has sufficient kinetic energy to penetrate skin. Upon leaving the nozzle of the gun the fluid forms micro droplets. As these droplets penetrate the skin they lose energy and begin to deviate from their original straight line. The maximum penetration of the fluid injected by this system is 3 cm and the droplets cone out to an approximate diameter of 2 cm. As might be expected, the deeper the fluid penetrates the less kinetic energy it has left, and it exhibits an increasing tendency to move along fascial planes in the body rather than to penetrate them. Early work in the development of the gun has shown that the peritoneum is an effective barrier to the spread of the fluid[1] and in the studies to be described the pleura appeared to behave in exactly the same way.

On theoretical grounds therefore, the gun could be expected to deliver fluid deep enough to reach the intercostal nerves but it should not penetrate the pleura and there should be no risk of causing pneumothorax. It was now necessary to test the gun to see if the theoretical possibility could be converted to reality. In all three studies were undertaken. The first to confirm that the risk of pneumothorax was negligible, the second to test whether analgesia was possible, and finally to ascertain whether intercostal nerve block could be produced with results comparable to those with conventional needle and syringe methods.

3. THE FIRST STUDY

The first research using the gun[2] was carried out in an attempt to define the possibility of risk to the pleura. The subjects were patients who had had open thoracotomy for bronchogenic carcinoma. Following the removal of the lung, with the chest open, an intercostal block using Lignocaine was performed by jet injection in such a position that the parietal pleura immediately deep to the injection site could be viewed from the inside as the injection was made. The sterile nozzle of the gun was pressed firmly into the intercostal space palpable on the exterior surface of the chest and 1 ml of Lignocaine was injected. As the injection was made the pleura deep to the injection site was noted to bulge slightly. The bulge produced by the injection had an approximate diameter of 2 cm which is in keeping with the known properties of the gun, and a height of possibly 2-3 mm. In all, 10 injections were made by this method and in every case the result was the same.

This study showed that the fluid behaved as predicted and reached a sufficient depth to reach the intercostal nerves. Furthermore, the parietal pleura acted as an effective barrier to the inner spread of the fluid. On no occasion was there any evidence of pleural damage and the risk of causing pneumothorax by this method must be regarded as negligible.

4. SECOND STUDY

To ascertain whether nerve block could, in fact, be produced by this method a clinical trial was now conducted.

The patients chosen were those who had had open-heart surgery 24 hours previously. These patients all had chest drains inserted at the time of operation and the drains themselves constituted a sort of pain which one might expect to be reduced if intercostal nerve block were performed. Furthermore, the drains themselves would protect should any pneumothorax be produced, and finally, these patients were subjected to serial chest X-rays for normal clinical reasons.

Before the block was performed the drains were aspirated to remove any blood from the thorax. This procedure is normally accompanied by some pain and the patients were asked to give that pain a score on a numerical analogue system where 1 represented no pain and 5 represented the most unbearable agony. Pinprick sensation over the relevant dermatomes was now tested and then intercostal nerve blocks were performed by jet injection at the relevant levels. At each intercostal space 1 millilitre of 0.5% bupivacaine + 1:200,000 adrenaline was injected. Thirty minutes later the patient had the drains aspirated again and the pinprick sensation was again tested for. They were asked to score their pain on the numerical scale again, and they were asked whether performing the block had been painless, had caused some discomfort or had been frankly painful. The results are shown in Table 1.

TABLE 1

Patient	Dose*	Pain levels** Pre-block	Pain levels** Post-block	Pinprick 0 min	Pinprick 30 min	Was block painful?
1	4	1	1	Sharp	Dull	No
2	8	2	1	Sharp	Dull	Some discomfort
3	5	3	1	Sharp	Dull	Some discomfort
4	5	3	2	Sharp	Dull	No
5***	3	–	–	Sharp	Dull	Some discomfort
6	5	3	3	Sharp	Dull	No
7	3	3	1.5	Sharp	Dull	No
8****	3	2	2	Sharp	Dull	Some discomfort
9****	5	3	3	Sharp	Dull	Some discomfort
	4	3	2	Sharp	Dull	Some discomfort

* In millilitre of 0.5% bupivacaine plus 1:200,000 adrenaline
** On numerical analogue (see text)
*** Co-operation poor, but some improvement subjectively
**** Bilateral drains, blocks separated by 5 hours

"Reproduced from Anaesthesia 1981, Vol. 36, p. 304-306 with kind permission of the Editor".

It is clear from this work that intercostal nerve block was, indeed, produced by jet injection and that the procedure was not unduly uncomfortable for the patients. However, it is quite clear that analgesia produced in this study was not complete. There are two reasons why this should be so. First, and possibly most importantly, the patients all had sources of pain which would not be amenable to relief by intercostal nerve block. Many had sternotomy wounds as well as visceral components to their pain. Secondly, the dose of local anaesthetic used was much smaller than would normally be given by the needle and syringe method.

None of the patients showed any evidence of pneumothorax and there were no demonstrable side-effects. However, the analgesia produced, although measurable, was relatively short-lived in the order of 3-4 hours and this again probably reflects the dose of local anaesthetic given.

These results were clearly sufficiently significant to warrant further work and it was our intention to perform intercostal nerve blocks by this method but using a higher dose of local anaesthetic. However, increasing the dose delivered was not so simple as it may seem. To increase the volume injected would involve either multiple injections of 1 ml or a delivery of a volume greater than 1 ml. At present there is no jet injection system on the market which can deliver a volume significantly greater than 1 ml. Furthermore, as can be seen from the results of this study, the injection did cause some discomfort in about 50% of the patients, and also the gas cylinders supplied would not run to more than 10 or 12 ml injections without having to be changed. Clearly, therefore, it was more practical to increase the concentration of local anaesthetic used so that the dose would approximate to that delivered by needle and syringe.

Unfortunately, concentrated local anaesthetics are potentially neurotoxic and so before embarking on study an exhaustive search of the literature was necessary to be sure that the higher concentration of bupivacaine which it was planned to use would not cause toxicity problems. The result of this search of the literature was 2% bupivacaine was found to carry a slight risk of neurotoxicity. In one study[3] solutions of bupivacaine of varying strength were painted directly onto the exposed sciatic nerves of rabbits and in one specimen out of eight, epineural thickening was produced with a 2% solution. No problems were encountered at concentrations lower than this and it was decided therefore to use 1.5% solution of bupivacaine for this work. This solution was specially prepared for the project by Messrs Duncan, Flockhart.

5. THIRD STUDY

In this study intercostal nerve block was used to provide analgesia inter-operatively and post-operatively for patients undergoing cholecystectomy. Previous work[4] has shown that intercostal nerve block is a useful analgesic supplement for this operation and in this study the jet injector was used to provide the block and the results were compared with conventional needle and syringe methods. Twenty patients about to have cholecystectomy were divided into two groups of similar age and general fitness, one of which was to receive an intercostal nerve block and the other would act as control. All patients received a premedication of 15 mgms papaveretum and 0.3 mgms of hyoscine. Anaesthesia was induced with "Althesin", relaxation produced with alcuronium, both given in appropriate dosage, and then the group who were about to have the intercostal block were turned into the left lateral position and 1 ml of 1.5% bupivacaine and 1:200,000 adrenaline was injected at each intercostal space from T4 to T11. The patient was now turned to the supine position and the operation performed using the right subcostal incision. Postoperatively, the patients were taken to the Recovery Room and the time from the start of the operation to the first request for analgesia was noted. Secondly, the total requirements of analgesia over the next 48 hours was compared with the control group. The results are shown in Table 2.

TABLE 2

	Mean time to first analgesia in the first 24 hours	Mean requirements of papaveretum in the first 24 hours
STUDY GROUP	12.1 hours	33 mgms
CONTROL GROUP	2.7 hours	69 mgms

"This is produced with the kind permission of the Editor of Anaesthesia" (To be published)

Two hours after the start of the operation 80% of the control group had requested analgesia, whereas only 10% of those who had received an intercostal block had done so. The results accord very well with those produced by Nunn[4].

Twenty four hours after the operation all the patients were tested for the return of pinprick sensation over the relevant dermatomes. There was no evidence of persistent analgesia and chest X-rays on the patient showed no cases of pneumothorax.

6. CONCLUSION

These studies have shown that intercostal nerve block is a feasible technique using jet injection. The results are very similar to those available using conventional needle and syringe. Furthermore, there appears to be no risk of pneumothorax associated with this technique.

Technically it is very easy to perform such a nerve block and requires no special training. However, two problems do remain. On two occasions while conducting this study, fine grit particles blocked the orifice of the gun and prevented effective utilisation of the technique, and secondly, the local anaesthetic solution used in the final study had to be made specially as it is not commercially available.

REFERENCES

1. McKenzie R, Shaffer WL. A safer method for paracervical block in therapeutic abortions. American Journal of Obstetrics and Gynaecology 1978; 130: 317-20
2. Seddon SJ and Doran BRH. Alternative method of intercostal blockade. Anaesthesia 1981; Vol. 36: p. 304-306
3. Selander D, Brattsand R, Lundborg G, Nordborg C and Olsson Y, Local anaesthetics: Importance of mode of application, concentration and adrenaline for appearance of nerve lesions. Acta Anaesthesiologica Scandinavia 1977; 21: p. 182
4. Nunn JF and Slavin J. Posterior intercostal nerve block for pain relief after cholecystectomy. Brit. J. of Anaesthesia 1980; 52: 253-259

THE MIXED LUMBAR-LUMBOSACRAL OR PSOASCOMPARTMENT BLOCK

J.T.A. KNAPE

1.   INTRODUCTION.

The contribution of regional anesthesia to the total number of anesthesias administered in the Netherlands and in Western Europe has increased considerably in the last few years. Although the statistics of my own small hospital cannot be considered to be representative, it is worth while to observe that the amount of regional anesthetics administered has increased from 0.3 to more than 25 % in the last decade.

Of the various regional blocks, however, not all blocks have gained a popularity to the same extent. Peripheral nerve blocks for instance, are less frequently administered than epidural or spinal blockades. Although peripheral nerve blocks may provide the safest form of anesthesia for a variety of surgical procedures, anesthesiologists are still reluctant to use them because of various reasons.

Peripheral nerve blocks on the upper extremity have gained a certain popularity. One of the important factors that have contributed to this popularity is the concept of the tubular peri-neurovascular sheath. The presence of this sheath of connective tissue enclosing the brachial plexus enables the anesthesiologist to block the radial, median, ulnar and musculocutaneous nerves arising from the brachial plexus, by the deposition of a local anesthetic within this perineural sheath by one injection, a so-called single needle technique. Five single needle techniques are most frequently used nowadays usually named after the inventor and the point of the needle-insertion:the supraclavicular (Kulenkampff[1] axillary (Hirschel[2] and Eriksson[3] subclavian perivascular (Winnie)[4] interscalene

(Winnie[5], and the infraclavicular approach described by Raj[6]
The relative ease to learn these techniques, the high success-
rate and the relative absence of discomfort for the patient
with these single needle techniques have all contributed to the
spread and acceptance of these procedures.

Peripheral nerve blocks on the lower extremity, however,
have never been very popular. A problem is that a blockade
of the four principal nerves to the lower extremity, the femoral
nerve, the lateral femoral cutaneous nerve, the obturator nerve
and the sciatic nerve can only be achieved by blocking each of
these nerves separately. Due to the anatomy in this region,
which is often not very simple, these procedures can be quite
laborious indeed.

The least inconvenient technique in this respect for the
patient is Winnies 3 in 1 block. By this single needle technique
in the inguinal region a blockade of the femoral, the lateral
femoral cutaneous and the obturator nerves can be accomplished.
These three nerves emerge from the lumbar plexus which is located
between the psoas major muscle ventrally and the quadratus
lumborum muscle dorsally. It should be realized that this
technique also has been based on the concept of a nerve plexus
covered by a tubular sheath of connective tissue, since digital
compression distal to the puncture site should aid in a rostral
spread of the anesthetic solution within the sheath. A
disadvantage is the necessity to block the sciatic nerve
separately.

An additional point against peripheral nerve blocks on the
lower extremity is that good alternatives can be offered to the
patient. In the hands of a skilfull anesthesiologist, epidural
and spinal anesthesia are reliable techniques, which are usually
not uncomfortable to the patient.
Yet this does not mean that a peripheral nerve blockade of
the lower extremity by one single injection of a local anesthetic
within the sheath around the lumbar and lumbosacral plexus
is impossible.

2. HISTORY

In the beginning of this century, when most of the techniques of regional anesthesia in current use were developed and refined, investigations have been carried out and published on regional anesthetic techniques of the lower extremity.

In 1915 Schlesinger[7] reported that the lumbar plexus could be blocked by one single paravertebral injection of a local anesthetic at L5-S1 for the first time:Für den Plexus lumbalis gibt es eine Stelle wo sämtliche Fasern desselben gemeinsam getroffen werden können. For the lumbar plexus there is a site where all its fibers together can be hit. He even remarked a similarity between the lumbar and the brachial plexus and observe analgesia in certain sacral nerves!

Degenhardt[8], 1926, described the excellent results of this technique combined with a sciatic block in 46 operations on the inguinal region and on the lower extremity.

After a long period of silence new interest in regional anesthesia of the lumbar plexus was aroused in the seventies. Winnie[9], 1973, describing his 3 in 1 block, suggested the possibility of a blockade of the lumbar plexus from a more centra site by injecting a larger volume of local anesthetic.

In 1976 Winnie[10] described his combined lumbosacral block and in the same year Cha en et al.[11] published their article on the posterior approach to the lumbar plexus, based on the fact that most of the branches of the lumbar plexus and some of the branche of the lumbosacral plexus supplying the thigh are found close to each other in the region of the fourth lumbar vertebra in what they call the "psoas-compartment".

Oddly enough sensory and motor blockade of the lower extremit were reported as a complication of other regional anesthetic techniques more than once. Feldman[12], 1975, stated that the inadvertent spread of a local anesthetic in the psoasmuscle sheath (proved by X-ray studies) could lead to a blockade of the adjacent somatic nerves, resulting in temporary pareses and analgesia of the lower extremity. Löfstrom[13], in the chapter

on sympathetic neural blockade of upper and lower extremities
in Cousins textbook "Neural Blockade" mentioned that a loss of
resistance is often obtained at a shallower level than the
sympathetic chain between the psoasmuscle and the quadratus
lumborum-muscle in the region of the transverse process. Placement
of solution will result in a lumbar plexus blockade, which is
highly undesirable if a neurolytic solution is employed.

The point of interest which cannot unequivocally be answered
from the literature is whether a blockade of the lumbar (L2-L4)
and the lumbosacral plexus (L4-S2) can be achieved by a posterior
approach with a single needle technique.

3.   CADAVER STUDIES.

We, especially my collegue Louis Richard, anesthesiologist
at St. Lambertus Hospital, Helmond, The Netherlands, therefore
did cadaverstudies. Dissection studies in bodies donated for the
purpose of medical science revealed in the first place a
macroscopically visible continuity between the lumbar plexus
(L2-L4) and the lumbosacral plexus (L4-S2). This positive finding
led us to investigate whether it would be possible to reach this
psoascompartment by a posterior approach. In our cadavers, of
course, we could not identify this compartment with the aid of
a nerve stimulator. However, identification of the psoascompartment with a loss-of-resistance technique using a
conventional 18-G epidural needle proved to be amazingly simple.
After the introduction of an epidural catheter 1 cm beyond the
tip of the needle, the needle was withdrawn and the catheter
secured with adhesive tape. Upon dissection of the body the
catheter was found to ly in the psoascompertment itself. Roentgen
contrast medium injected via the epidural - or I had better say
the psoascompertment catheter in another cadaver before dissection
- was found in the psoascompartment down to the S2-level in the
pelvis over its brim. It seems therefore possible to reach the
psoascompartment, comprising roots of L2 to S2,with a single
needle technique by a posterior approach.

4. ANATOMIC CONSIDERATIONS

The lower limb, and especially its anterior and lateral upper parts, is mainly innervated by the nerve branches of the lumbar, the lumbosacral and to a lesser degree the sacral plexus.

The lumbar plexus supplies the innervation of the anterior part by the femoral nerve and its derivatives (L2-L4), the medial aspects of the lower limb by the obturator (L2-L4) and branches of the femoral and genitofemoral nerve (L2-L4) and the lateral thigh by the lateral femoral cutaneous nerve (L2-L3) .

The lumbosacral plexus provides nerve supply to the anterior and lateral posterior parts of the calf and foot, and gives off branches to the posterior part of the lower limb, which is innervated mainly by the sciatic nerve (L4-S3). This nerve finds its origin mainly in the sacral, and to a lesser degree in the lumbosacral plexus.

The anterior primary rami of the paravertebral nerves L2-L4 form the part of the lumbar plexus responsible for the innervatio of the lower limb. After supplying the psoas and quadratus lumborum muscle with motor fibres, this lumbar plexus, already branching into major components like the femoral and obturator nerves, lies in an anatomic compartment at the lower lumbar level between the psoas muscle and its fascia anteriorly, the periosteu: of the lumbar vertebrae medially, the transverse processes, their common ligaments and the fascia of the quadratus lumborum muscle posteriorly and the conjoint fasciae of the quadratus lumborum and psoas major muscles laterally. From the lumbar plexus the femoral nerve emerges posterolaterally and the obturator nerve anteromedially to the psoas major muscle. Medioposteriorly to the obturator nerve a fusion of branches of L4 and L5 descends to for: the lumbosacral trunk. This lumbosacral trunk enters the pelvis and forms the sacral plexus with the ventral rami of the first, second and third sacral nerves and part of the ventral ramus of the fourth sacral nerve.

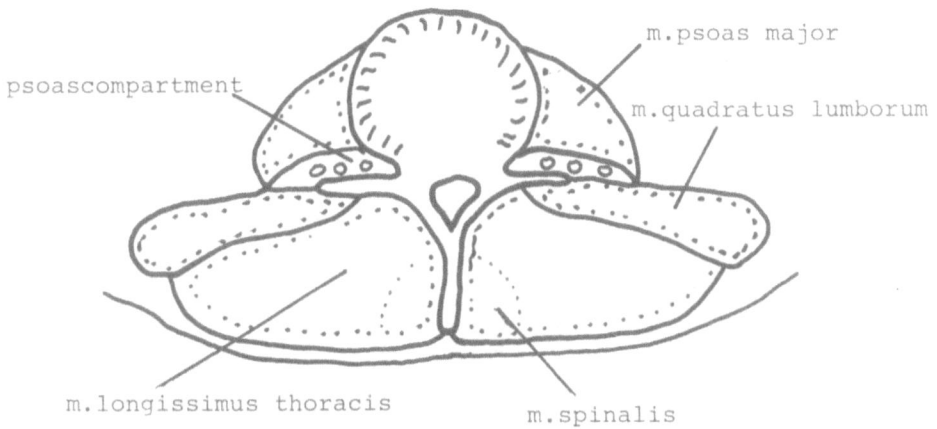

The above mentioned lateral cutaneous femoral nerve, the
genitofemoral nerve, the femoral nerve, the obturator nerve and
the lumbosacral plexus can be found in close proximity in the
psoascompartment at the level between the transverse processus
L4-L5.

5. TECHNIQUE.
    After the usual inspection of the resuscitation equipment
and the insertion of an intravenous cannula, the patient is
placed in the lateral decubitus position on the side not to be
operated upon. A line is drawn connecting the superior borders
of both iliac crests. At a point about 3 to 4 cm caudal and
4 to 5 cm lateral from the midline the skin is infiltrated with
4 ml 0.5 % lidocaine under aseptic conditions. A 20-G spinal
needle is inserted perpendicular to the skin and directed slightly
medially. A glass syringe is attached to the needle and with
the loss-of-resistance technique the psoascompartment can be
identified, usually about 6 to 8 cm beneath the skin surface.
If the fifth transverse process is encountered the needle is
redirected to reach the psoascompartment. After carefull
aspiration 30 to 50 ml of a suitable local anesthetic like for
instance bupivacaine 0.375 to 0.5 % is injected in the psoascompartment,where relatively few vessels are found in contrast

to the brachial plexus, after a test dose, in a course of two
minutes and the needle is removed.

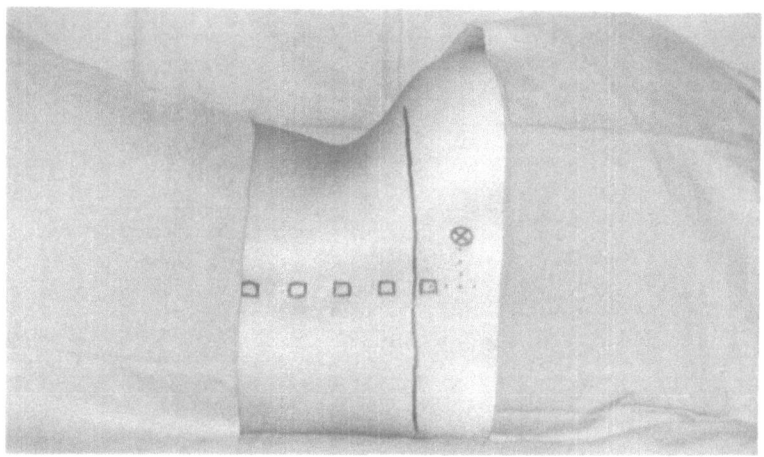

An 18-G epidural needle is employed in case a catheter
technique is preferred. Identification of the psoascompartment
with the aid of a nerve stimulator is also a possibility.
The anesthesiologist, however, should not be misled by flexion
of the hip when the psoasmuscle is stimulated directly. He should
be certain to observe contractions of the adductor muscles of
the thigh.

6. INDICATIONS.
    The psoascompartment block can be applied for anesthesia
of the lower limb, for for instance vascular surgery and
orthopaedic[14] operations like surgery on the hip (hip prosthesis,
total hip replacement surgery) and osteosynthesis of the tibia
and of the ankle. The technique is not suitable for surgery
in the inguinal region. We have experienced some difficulties
in surgery on the knee, probably because of the contribution
of the sciatic nerve to the innervation of the posterior surface
and the deep structures of the knee. In our hospital the techniqu
is employed with great success for anesthesia in total hip
replacement surgery, an operation frequently performed. Combined
with a minimal amount of an inhalational anesthetic in the
elderly patient, this technique provides profound analgesia in

the lower limb during surgery but also in the postoperative
period in a quickly alert patient.

Cardiovascular stability is excellent and superior to epidural
or spinal anesthesia since the area where vasodilatation occurs
is limited to one limb. Blood loss is similar to blood loss
under epidural analgesia and less than with neurolept anesthetic
techniques. The technique is very usefull for patients with
malformations of the lumbar spine, like in reumatoïd arthritis,
where a spinal or epidural approach is not possible.

It must be concluded that a peripheral nerve block of the
lower extremity by a single injection with a local anesthetic
is a possibility. Whether the psoascompartment block will gain
the same popularity as the plexus blocks of the upper extremity
remains to be seen. The technique deserves more interest and
research than it has received up till now.

AKNOWLEDGEMENT.

The author wishes to thank Louis C. Richard, anesthesiologist,
St. Lambertus Hospital, Helmond, for his substantial aid and
advises.

REFERENCES

1.Kulenkampff D. 1912, Die Anaesthesierung des Plexus brachialis.
v.Bruns' Beitr.,Bd.79, Heft 3.
2. Hirschel B. 1911, Die Anwendung der Lokalanaesthesie bei
grösseren Operationen an Brust und Thorax. (Mammakarzinom,
Thorakoplastik) Münchener Med. Wochenschrift,10: 497.
3. Eriksson E, Skarby HG. 1962, A simplified method of axillary
block. Nord Med, 68:1325.
4. Winnie AP, Collins VJ. 1964, The subclavian perivascular
technique of brachial plexus anesthesia. Anesthesiology,25:353.
5. Winnie AP.1970, Interscalene brachial plexus block. Anesth.
Analg. 49:455.
6. Raj PP, Montgomery SJ, Nettles D, Jenkins MT.1973, Infraclavicular brachial plexus block - A new approach. Anesth. Analg.
52: 897.
7. Schlesinger A. 1915, Über Versuche den Plexus lumbalis zu
anästhesieren. Zentralblatt für Chirurgie,22:385.
8. Degenhardt H. 1926. Die Leitungsanesthesie des Plexus lumbalis.
Zentralblatt für Chirurgie,25:1570.
9. Winnie AP, Ramamurthy S, Durrani Z. 1973, The inguinal
paravascular technique of lumbar plexus anesthesia.:The 3 in 1
block. Anesth. Analg. 52:989.

10. Winnie AP.1976, Plexus anesthesia. In ASA refresher course lectures, 126:1.
11. Chayen D, Nathan H, Chayen M. 1976, The Psoas compartment block. Anesthesiology, 45:95.
12. Feldman SA, Yeung ML.1975, Treatment of intermittent claudication. Lumbar paravertebral block. Anaesthesia,30:174.
13. Löfstrom JB, Cousins MJ. 1980, Sympathetic neural blockade of upper and lower extremities. In: Cousins MJ, Bridenbaugh PO. Neural Blockade. Lippincott Company, Philadelphia, 1980, p.355.
14. Bernstein RL. 1980, Anesthesia for total hip replacement. in: Zauder HL ed. Anesthesia for orthopaedic surgery. Davis, Philadelphia, 1980, p. 67.

TRANSSACRAL BLOCK

H.U. GERBERSHAGEN
D.H. FROHNEBERG
Ch. PANHANS
H. WAISBROD

The sacral nerves can be blocked, a. by injecting a local anesthetic solution into the individual posterior sacral foramen, b. by depositing the solution close to the anterior sacral foramen and c. by performing a caudal block.

In 1913 the injection into the transsacral canal (representing the fused transverse processes of the sacral vertebrae) has been termed t r a n s s a c r a l   b l o c k by its initiator Danis (10). The presacral deposition of local anesthetic solution, first described by Braun (5), a German surgeon in 1918, was called p r e s a c r a l   or p a r a s a c r a l   block.

Danis (10) realized, of course, that by injecting the local anesthetic solution deep into the transsacral canal he also anesthetized the sacral nerve fibers close to the presacral foramen and within the spinal canal (thus achieving a transsacral and presacral blockade as well as a caudal block. The volume dependancy of this block procedure in obvious).

TECHNIQUE

The four sacral foramina are about one centimeter in diameter and three of them (S2-S4) are located on a line 1,5 cm lateral to the midline.

As for all regional anesthetic procedures an intravenous catheter is placed. The patient is asked either to lie prone with a pillow under his hips so that the sacrum is elevated and tilted to a 45-degree angle to the table or to sit on a special urological chair.

The posterior superior iliac spine is palpated and the skin marked 1,5 cm laterally and caudally to this palpable area. A skin wheal is raised and a 6 cm long, needle, 22-24g (=0,70-0,55 mm in diameter), is inserted unattached to the syringe. If the needle does not at once enter the second sacral foramen, one has to feel about with needle ("hunt and peck-method" (17), the needle is slightly withdrawn and reinserted several times in a systematic fanwise direction (2)). When the foramen has been located a line parallel to the midline is drawn through the point where the needle supposedly contacted the foramen. The third and fourth sacral foramina are each situated some 1,5 cm caudally on this line, and the fifth sacral nerve (rarely emerging from a separate foramen) will be found 1,5 cm caudally to the fourth sacral foramen. The first sacral foramen is located some 2 cm cranially and 2 cm laterally to the second sacral foramen.

We never insert the needle more than 1 cm into the first and second transsacral canal or 0,5 cm into the third and fourth. We inject small volumes only (1-5 ml).

The posterior primary divisions of the sacral nerves are easily blocked by slowly injecting 1-2 ml of local anesthetic solution. For surgical procedures up to 10 ml per canal have been advocated (17,18).

The injection of large volumes of local anesthetics will cause a spread of the solution to adjacent roots and into the spinal canal.

In table 1 the lengths of needles, the volumes of local anesthetics and neurolytics are summerized.

Table 1: Transsacral Block: needle length, volumes of
          local anesthetics and neurolytics

	S1	S2	S3	S4	S5
length of needle (cm)	6-8	6	4	4	3-4
volume of l.a.* (ml)	3-4	2-3	2	1,5-2	1,5
volume of ethanol (50%) (ml)	2	2	1-2	1-2	1
volume of 6% aqueous phenol (ml)	2-3	2-3	2	2	1,5

Figure 1, taken from Pauchet ([18]) emphasizes the variable
thickness of the subcutaneous tissues overlying the posterior sacral foramina, the variable depth of the transsacral
canal and the length of the needle.

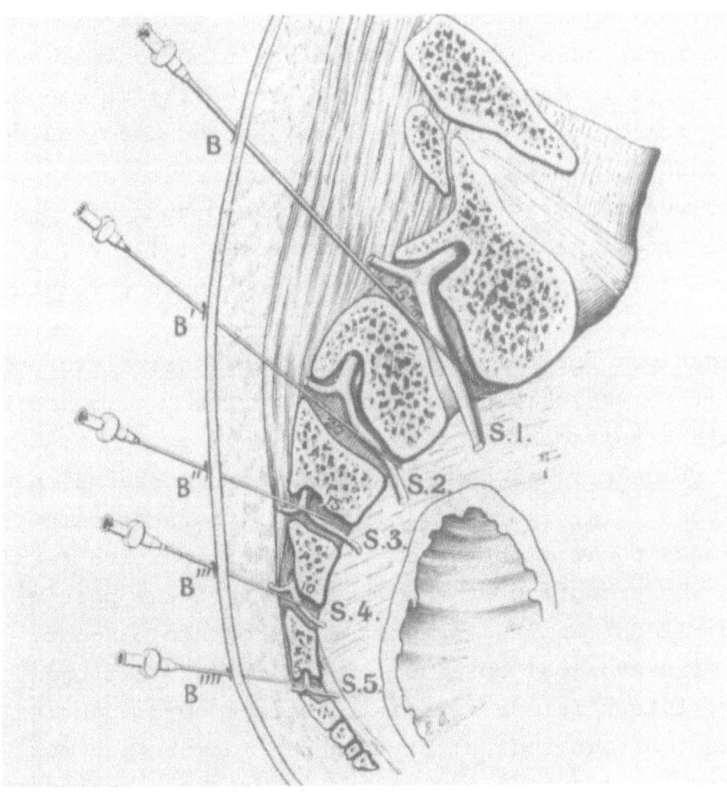

Often paresthesias are elicited when entering the canal.
We use nerve stimulators in order to be sure that the area
of the radiating sensation corresponds with that supplied
by the nerve (27). Periosteally - elicited dysesthesias
may otherwise mislead the physician. The use of fluorosco-
pic techniques in the localization of the posterior sacral
foramina has already been advocated by Meirowski and cowor-
kers (15) in 1969 and can certainly be recommended. This
is in particular true for the injection of a single sacral
nerve with phenol or ethanol.

Indications for surgical procedures

Reviewing the extensive literature on transsacral anesthesia it becomes obvious that this block technique has had
merits in the pioneering days of regional anesthesia. Today,
it is obsolete for surgical anesthesia. In 1916 Härtel (10),
a great regional anesthesiologist, wrote in his excellent
textbook on local anesthesia "transsacral block compared to
other procedures is cumbersome. The person using it can be
compared to someone who enters a house, having wide and open
doors, through a window" (10).

For many years American authors advocated to perform
transsacral blocks along with a caudal block (12,17   ).
With todays local anesthetics this combination is obsolete,
too.

A. Indications for pelvic pain and functional disturbances

Chronic rectal, vesical, prostatic and perineal pain has been
treated with transsacral blocks (2, 14, 22, 26   ). Cancer
pain, in particular, has been managed with transsacral neurolytic blocks (8, 13,20,21). In our 15 years of pain clinic experience we have observed short-lived positive results
only, with the exception of the management of the painful
contracted bladder and the inhibited neurogenic bladder.

Tumors, intravesical obstruction, radiation, estrogen
deficiency, interstitional cystitis, spinal cord injuries
and disease, foreign bodies, psychogenic factors and most
inflammatory lesions of the bladder can cause frequency,

urgency, dysuria and induce urge incontinence, reflex incontinence (upper motor neuron lesion) and a reduction in
bladder capacity. This symptomatology incapacitates the patient and often patients become "bladder cripples". These
patients have been managed primarily with pharmacologic
agents (anticholonergic and spasmolytic drugs) and surgical procedures (prolonged bladder distention under anesthesia, bladder denervation, selective rhizotomies (7, 19),
surgical urinary diversion, bladder augmentation, cystolysis.)
The results have been poor to fair.

Uninhibited bladder activity is mediated by the sacral
reflex arc and can be abolished by caudal anesthesia (4,
11,15). Local anesthetic block of the involved sacral roots
was reported to effectively reduce the incapacitating factors (7, 9, 15, 16, 20, 21, 22, 28, 32).

Since the early 70's we have been interested in upper
motor neuron lesions. Thus, we did, like many other rese-
archers, study the innervation of the bladder and its sphinc-
ter by sequental diagnostic sacral blocks with 1,0 and
2,0 ml of lidocain (1%) with the patient in the sitting
position. If there was no significant effect noticable
by urodynamic measurements and urgency not changed according to patient's report, the next sacral nerve was blocked.
The sequence was changed from unilateral blocks i.e. blok-
king the nerves from S2 to S5 on one side to S2, S3, S4
on both sides a.s.o.

Prospective study in patients with upper motor neuron
lesions
In spite of the great variations of detrusor innervation in
individual patients we started a prospective study on bilateral S3 and S4 blocks. The same protocol was used from
1976 until 1981. 27 patients were selected who had been un-
sucessfully treated by conservative methods. Control measurements of urodynamic functions were obtained in the sitting
patient. Then needle electrodes were placed into the third

and fourth transsacral foramina bilaterally. The paresthesias reported were in the perineal and paraanal regions.
A total of 5 ml of bupivacaine (0,5%) were injected bilaterally. 10 and 90 minutes after the injection the urodynamic examinations were repeated.

Results

An increased bladder capacity was determined in21 of our
27 patients with bladder instability (range 1o to 50%;
19 patients had increased bladder volumes at first desire
to void (range 1o to 35%) within the first 120 minutes.
After the bupivacaine blocks 10 of 27 patients had reduced
frequentcy, but still some urgency, for 4 - 7 weeks. In 17
patients the symptoms were essentially unchanged after
wearing off of the blockade.

8 patients with good block responses after 3 weeks un-
terwent bilateral S3 and S4 blocks with phenol (2ml of 6%
aqueous phenol per transsacral foramen). In 2 patients we
recorded an increased bladder capacity and a diminished
detrusor instability lasting longer than 7 months. 4 patients reported definite subjective improvement even
though the urodynamic investigations showed no significant changes.

Advantages and disadvantages of transsacral blocks in unstable bladder disease

This simple technique is non-invasive and inexpensive. It
can be repeated several times. Short term results are
satisfactory and positive psychological effects are often
observed.

The main disadvantages of the method are its unpredictable therapeutic effect, the relative short effective
duration, even after neurolytic blockade, the transient
sensory loss in the S3 and S4 segments, and occassionally
residual urine.

Nevertheless, regional anesthesiologists should be fa-
miliar with transsacral block and offer their help to patients suffering from detrusor instability. Diagnostic

blocks before the performance of phenol blocks and especially of selective rhizotomy are most important.

    B. <u>Indications for coccygeal and sacroiliac pain</u>

Blocks of the fifth sacral nerves have been used for the
treatment of coccygodynia (12, 26). Our results with
local anesthetic and/or phenol- and alcohol blocks have
regularly been poor.

    We developed a new method of treating pain of sacro-
iliac joint origin in 1982. The innervation of the dorsal
side of the sacroiliac joint has its origin in the first
and second sacral nerves (23). In patients suffering
from sacrolumbar instability accompanied by sacroiliac
joint arthropathy it is often difficult to evaluate the
causative lesion. It has been our experience in 55 patients
that diagnostic blocks of the first, second and, in addition, the third sacral nerves are valuable in these patients. This is especially true since in the majority of
these patients diagnostic intraarticular injection cannot
be performed due to arthrotic changes. In 18 patients, in
whom 2-3 diagnostic sacral nerve blocks eliminated their
typical pain patterns temporarily we performed controlled
thermocoagulations of the S1-S3 nerves (radiofrequency
lesions) using RAY-needles (Radionics, Boston). The short-
term results (6-18 months) have been encouraging; some 50%
of patients did require no further treatment.

    <u>Complications of transsacral blocks</u>

Provided that principles of regional blocks are observed,
complications should not occur. Complications will be observed if aspiration tests (blood, cerebrospinal fluid)
are not performed, too large amounts of local anesthetics
or too large volumes of neurolytics are injected,or if
an intravenous indwelling needle has not been placed.

REFERENCES

1. Adriani J. 1967. Labat's Regional Anesthesia. Saunders, Philadelphia
2. Bonica JJ. 1953. The Management of Pain. Lea & Febiger, Philadelphia
3. Bors E, Comarr AE. 1979. Neurological Urology. University, Park Press, Baltimore
4. Bradley WE, Teague GT. 1968. The pelvic ganglia. J.Urol. 100:649
5. Braun H. 1918. Praesakral-Anästhesie. Zbl.Gynäk. 42
6. Erikson E. (ed) 1979. Illustrated Handbook in Local Anaesthesia. Lloyd-Luke, London
7. Gargour GW, Toczek SK, McCulloch DC. 1973. Selective sacral rootlet section for experimental detrusor inhibition. J.Neurosurg. 38:494
8. Goffen BS. 1982. Transsacral block. Anesth.Analg.61: 623
9. Green JF, Grennell H, Awad SA. 1974. Selective sacral nerve blocks in the management of "unhibited neurogenic bladder". Canad.Anaesth.Soc.J. 21:417
10. Härtel FC. 1916. Die Lokalanästhesie. F.Enke, Stuttgart
11. Heimburger RF, Freeman LW, Wilde NJ. 1948. Sacral nerve innervation of the human bladder. J.Neurosurgery 5:154
12. Killian H. 1973. Lokalanästhesie und Lokalanästhetika. G. Thieme, Stuttgart
13. Labat GS. 1928. Regional Anesthesia. Saunders, Philadelphia
14. Mandel F. 1947. Paravertebral block. Grune & Stratton, New York
15. Meirowski AM. 1969. The management of chronic interstitial cystitis by differential sacral neurotomy. J.Neurosurg. 30: 604
16. Moulder MK, Meirowski AM. 1956. The management of Hunner's ulcer by differential sacral neurotomy, Preliminary report. J.Urology 75:261
17. Moore DC. 1975. Regional block. Ch.C.Thomas, Springfield, Ill.
18. Pauchet-Sourdat-Labouré. 1917. Anesthésie Régional. Doin, Paris
19. Rockwold GL, Bradley WE, Chou SN. 1973. Differential sacral rhizotomy in the treatment of neurogenic bladder dysfunction. J.Neurosurg. 38,748
20. Rockwold GL, Bradley WE, Chou SN. 1974. Effect of sacral nerve blocks on the function of the urinary bladder in humans. J.Neurosurg. 409,83
21. Rockwold GL, Bradley WE. 1977. The use of sacral nerve blocks in the evaluation and treatment of neurologic bladder disease. J.Urology 118:415
22. Simon DL, Carron H, Rowlingson JC. 1982. Treatment of bladder pain with transsacral nerve block. Anesth.Analg. 61:46
23. Solonen KA. 1957. The sacroiliac joint in the light of anatomical, roentgenological and clinical studies. E. Munksgaard, Copenhagen

24. Sherwood-Dunn B. 1922. Regional Anesthesia (victor Pauchet's Technique) Davis, Philadelphia
25. Susset JG, Zinner N, Archimbaud JP. 1974. Differential sacral blocks and selective neurotomy in the treatment of incomplete upper motor neuron lesion. Urol.int. 29: 236
26. Swerdlow M. Peripheral nerve blocks. In:Lipton, S.1977. Persistent pain: Modern methods of treatment.Academic Press, London
27. Theiss D, Robbel G, Theiss M, Gerbershagen HU. 1977. Experimentelle Bestimmung einer optimalen Elektrodenanordnung zur elektrischen Nervenstimul-tion. Anaesthesist 26: 411
28. Torrens MJ, Griffith HB. 1976. Management of the uninhibitated bladder by selective sacral neurectomy. J.Neurosurg. 44:176
29. Susset JG, Pinheiro J, Otton P, Brindle F, Bertrand G. 1969. Phenolisation et neurotomie sélective fans la traitment de la dysfonction vesicale neurogène par lésion centrale incomplète. J.Urol.Nephrol.Suppl. 12, 75:502
30. Torrens MJ. 1974. The effect of selective sacral nerve blocks on vesical and urethral function. J.Urology 112:204
31. Van Erbs. 1924. Die transsakrale Anästhesie in der Geburtshilfe. Zentralorgan ges. Chir. 32:76
32. Westgate HD. 1970. Selective percutaneous sacral root blockade with phenol in neurovesial dysfunktion.Canad. Anaesth.Soc.J. 17:456

REGIONAL BLOCK IN CHILDREN

O. SCHULTE-STEINBERG

Regional anaesthesia in children is nothing new. As the following list shows it dates back up to 75 years. Pioneers of techniques were

1908	Grey	Spinal anaesthesia (7)
1920	Farr	Brachial plexus blockade (4)
1933	Campbell	Caudal epidural anaesthesia (2)
1936	Sievers	Lumbar epidural anaesthesia (12)
1971	Isakob	Thoracic epidural anaesthesia (8)

There are important anatomical differences between the child and the adult. They are shown in Table 1.

Table 1

Anatomical differences in children and adults
of importance in regional anaesthesia

	Neonate	Infant	Small Child	Older Child	Adult
Postion of lower end of spinal cord	L3		L1 at 12 mths		L1
Position of lower end of dural sac	S4 (one case)		S2		S2
CSF per kg	4 ml	4 ml	3 ml	2 ml	2 ml
Condition of epidural fat	loose	loose	loose	+ loose 7-8 years	firmly packed

It might be added that the cardio-vascular system of children is considerably more stable than in the adult.

The approach to regional anaesthesia in children has to be different from the adult, i.e. children require basal anaesthesia for almost all procedures including those where normally paraesthesias would be required like peripheral nerve blocks. The use of electrical nerve stimulators obviate the need for patient cooperation. When these preconditions are observed the entire spectrum of regional blocks may be weighted a little differently in children. Of course it also depends on the individual anaesthetist. However, it may be said that subarachnoid and lumbar epidural blocks enjoy only limited popularity, just the same as peripheral nerve blocks on the lower extremity. The caudal epidural route offers itself with its intriguing technical simplicity both for single shot and continuous techniques to replace the just mentioned methods.

Dosage: local anaesthetic agents used in children have to be carefully calculated on mg per kg body weight basis. Table 2 gives some details of doses.

Table 2

Local anaesthetic agents and doses in children

Agent	Topical use		Injection	
	Concentration (%)	Dose (mg/kg)	Plain solution dose (mg/kg)	Dose with epinephrine (mg/kg)
Lidocaine	2-10	3	5	7
Mepivacaine		5	5	7
Prilocaine			5-7	7-9
Chloroprocaine and procaine			7	10
Bupivacaine			2	2
Etidocaine			3	3-4
Dibucaine	0.2-0.5	1	subarachnoid use only	2
Cocaine	3-10	2		
Amethocaine (Tetracaine)	0.5-2	1	1.5 subarachnoid use only	1.5

Spinal anaesthesia is used relatively infrequent in children. Table 3 gives some details on drugs and doses. For lidocaine the influence of the varying CSF volumes on the dosage have been worked out in more detail. Such detailed information on tetracaine was not available. The technique in children - apart from basal anaesthesia - does not differ much from the procedure in the adult. A 5 cm 25 gauge needle is used.

Table 3

Recommended dosages for spinal anaesthesia in children

Expected duration of anaesthesia	Agent	Dose
Up to 45 minutes	5% hyperbaric lidocaine	Up to 3 years of age 2 mg/kg 3-10 years decreasing doses down to 1 mg/kg
45-90 minutes	1% tetracaine plus 10% glucose	1 mg per year of age in exceptionally small children 0.2 mg/kg
100-200 minutes	1% tetracaine plus 10% glucose containing 2 mg phenylephrine in 1 ml	As above

As compiled from Gouveia M.A.: Rev. Bras. Anest. 4, 503-511, 1970 and Berkowitz S, and Green B.A. Anesthesiology 12, 376-387, 1951 (6) (1)

Lumbar epidural anaesthesia is practiced in some centres. The dosage may be calculated in the same manner as it has been found for caudal epidurals i.e. 0.1 ml per segment per year of age. (10) (11)

The technique relies - like in the adult - on the loss of resistance test either with the 18 gauge Tuohy needle or - as it is also done - with a butterfly needle with an extension tubing.

The caudal approach of the epidural space both for single injections or with continuous techniques for higher dermatomes appears to be the quicker and safer method and is gaining popularity. Fig. 1 and 2 show the angulation of the needle as it pierces the skin and the sacral ligament until it is arrested by the anterior table of the sacrum. The epidural space has thus been entered. Following the test dose containing adrenaline to exclude an intravascular position of the needle opening - manifested by changes in pulse rate and extrasystoles seen in the ECG - the calculated dose for the single shot technique may be given. However, for the continuous method with an ordinary plastic intravenous needle this has to be introduced into the caudal canal with the guide needle about 1-2 cm once it has contacted the posterior table of the sacrum. The plastic sheath alone is advanced a

35

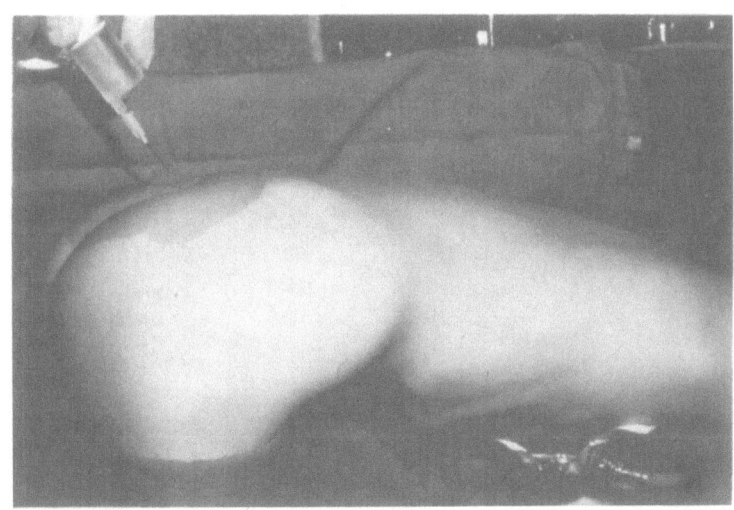

Fig. 1 **Caudal epidural blockade in the child.** This
photograph shows the needle insertion with the child
in the lateral postion. The drapes and the second
hand steadying the needle have been removed to show
the angulation. (Schulte-Steinberg, O.: Neural
blockade for pediatric surgery. In: Neural Blockade.
Cousins, M.J. and Bridenbaugh, P.O. (eds) J.B.
Lippincott Company, Philadelphia 1980)

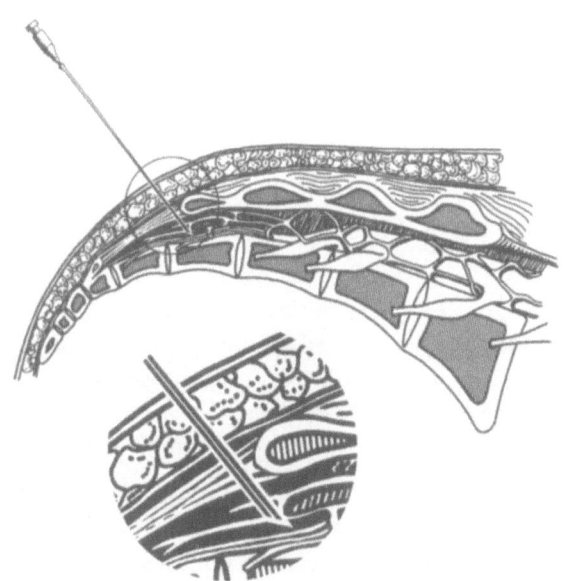

Fig. 2 (Schulte-Steinberg, O.: Neural blockade for pediatric
surgery. In: Neural Blockade. Cousins, M.J. and
Bridenbaugh, P.O. (eds) J.B. Lippincott Company,
Philadelphia 1980)

little further. Fig. 3 shows the plastic sheath in place and the catheter being measured prior to its introduction.

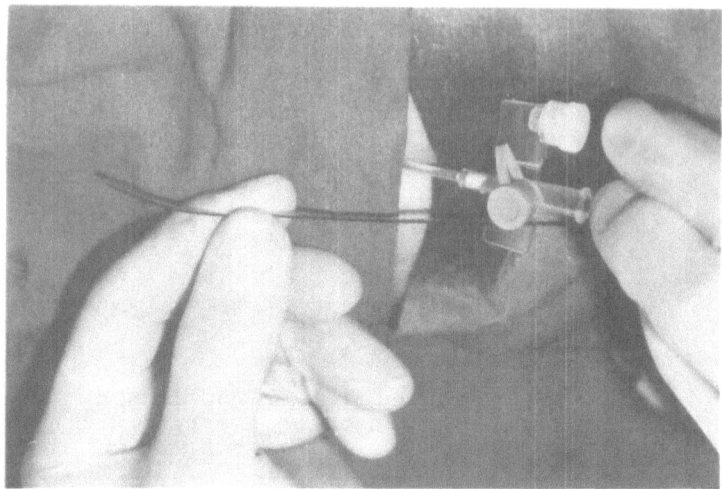

Fig. 3   Continuous caudal epidural blockade in the child. The plastic sheath is inserted into the caudal canal. After palpatory orientation of the iliac crests the catheter is measured for length.

Fig. 4 after this. The catheter can be advanced with great ease as far as the upper lumbar vertebrae. It is now used as an ordinary lumbar epidural anaesthetic, only that the catheter originates from the sacral hiatus. The dosage has been discussed before.

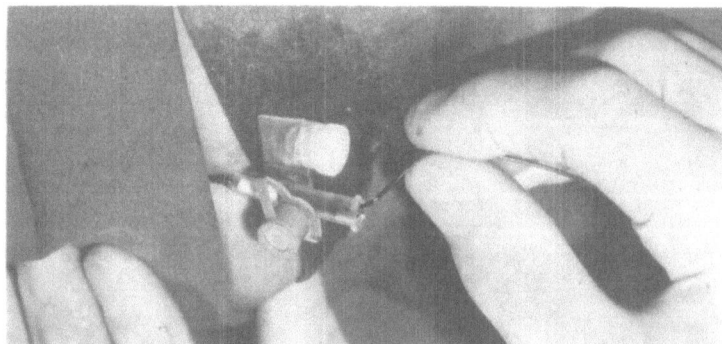

Fig. 4   Continuous caudal epidural blockade in the child. This photograph shows the measured length of the catheter after insertion without meeting any resistance.

It can be seen in more detail in Fig. 5 and 6. The continuous technique even permits its use for upper abdominal
procedures in combination with very light general anaesthesia
and intubation and avoidance of muscle relaxants. Other advantages are reduced blood loss and analgesia lasting into
the immediate postoperative period resulting in a tranquil
patient with less vomiting and a better chance for early oral
fluid intake after caudal blockade.

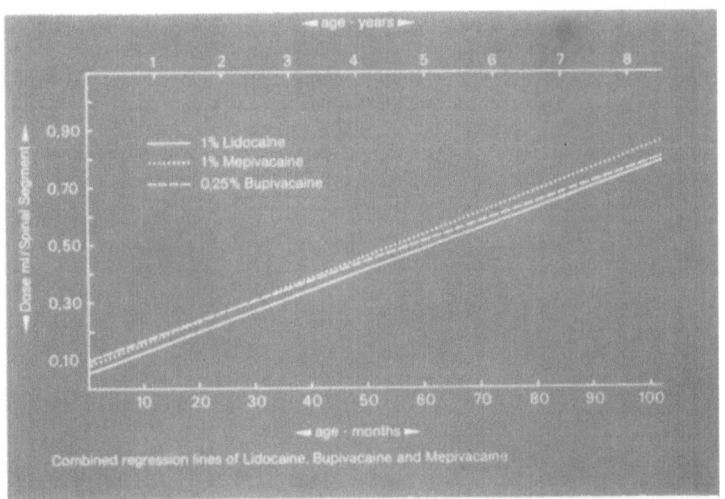

Fig. 5   Caudal epidural blockade in the child. Segmental dose
          requirements of lidocaine, mepivacaine and
          bupivacaine are related to age. (Schulte-Steinberg,
          O.: Neural blockade for pediatric surgery. In: Neural
          Blockade. Cousins, M.J. and Bridenbaugh, P.O. (eds)
          J.B. Lippincott Company, Philadelphia 1980)

Complications are essentially the same as in the adult.

Peripheral nerve blocks are mostly limited to the upper
extremity. While all peripheral blocks on the legs can be
done analgesia of the lower extremities is very simply and
securely achieved by caudal epidurals as mentioned before.
Therefore little need arises for peripheral blocks. The only
block procedure of the lower extremity distinguishing itself
apart from the caudal block is the "3 in 1" block. This is a
very useful and simple way to obtain analgesia in the child
with a fractured leg. It can even be performed at the scene
of an accident to permit painfree immobilization and trans-
portation.

For the upper extremity all approaches of the brachial
plexus are possible. Again they will mostly be preceeded by
basal anaesthesia and the plexus can be located with the
electrical nerve stimulator. One has to keep in mind - and
this applies in particular to the supraclavicular techniques

Table 4. Guide to Determination of Volume for Perivascular Anesthesia

Age (years)	Male Height (cm)	Male Volume (ml)	Female Height (cm)	Female Volume (ml)	Formula to Determine Volume (ml)	Concentration Lidocaine, Mepivacaine	Concentration Bupivacaine
Birth	53	4	50	4			
1	76	6	76	6			
2	91	7	91	7	$\dfrac{Height}{12.5}$	0.7-0.8	0.1875
3	101	8	101	8			
4	109	9	109	9			
5	116	12	114	11			
6	124	12.5	121	12	$\dfrac{Height}{10.3}$	0.8-0.9	0.25
7	132	14	129	12.5			
8	137	14	134	13			
9	142	18.5	139	18			
10	147	19	146	19			
11	152	20	152	20			
12	157	21	160	21	$\dfrac{Height}{7.7}$	0.9-1	0.25
13	165	22	165	22			
14	172	23	167	22			
15	177	23	167	22			
16	180	25	167	22.5			

(Data from Winnie, A.P.: Interscalene brachial plexus block. Anesth. Analg. (Cleve), 49:455,1970)

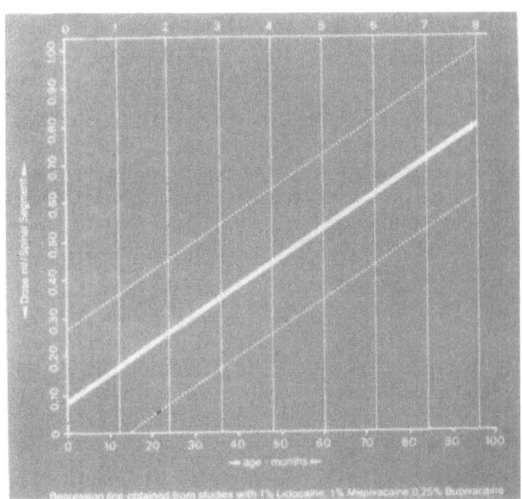

Fig. 6 Caudal epidural blockade in the child. Segmental dose
        requirements are related to age for 1 per cent
        lidocaine, 1 per cent mepivacaine, and 0.25 per cent
        bupivacaine. Computer-fitted regression line with 95
        per cent confidence limits. (Schulte-Steinberg, O.:
        Neural blockade for pediatric surgery. In: Neural
        Blockade. Cousins, M.J. and Bridenbaugh, P.O. (eds)
        J.B. Lippincott Company, Philadelphia 1980)

but also to the axillary approach - that all the structures
are much more superficial in children. Deeper penetration of
the needle will only result in failures and unnecessary
complications. The landmarks and techniques do not significantly differ from the adult. Local anaesthetic solutions
used are 0.75%-1% lidocaine or mepivacaine and 0.125-0.25%
bupivacaine.

Table 4 is taken from Winnie's work. It illustrates the
volumes used for interscalene brachial plexus blocks. (13)

For supraclavicular blocks the doses of local anaesthetic
agents are calculated not to exceed 3-5 mg/kg of lidocaine or
mepivacaine or 1.5 mg/kg of bupivacaine. The technique used

here is the "Short Needle Technique" described by Fortin. (5)
It avoids contact with the first rib.

The axillary approach of the brachial plexus is probably
the most popular one in children. But there really is no
reason for this absolute preference since the level of the
brachial plexus is largely dictated by the site of the surgical intervention. Again the technique of the axillary block
is not much different from the adult. The dosages of local
anaesthetics have been evaluated by Eriksson (3) and Niesel
(9) as shown in table 5.

Table 5

Axillary brachial plexus block volumes
equipotent to one per cent prilocaine

Age (years)	Volume (ml)
1-3	6-9
4-6	9-11
7-9	14-20
10-12	21-25
13-15	28-35

Intravenous regional anaesthesia also has a place in pae-
diatric work and it is best combined with basal anaesthesia,
particularly in the younger age group. The local anaesthetic
agent used is prilocaine at a dosage of 3-5 mg/kg of the 0.5%
solution. The youngest child who reportedly received an intravenous regional block was 3 years of age. The tourniquet
pressures used are 180-240 torr for the upper extremity and
350-500 torr for the lower.

In summary it can be stated that regional anaesthesia in
children often helps to avoid some of the dangers and difficulties encountered with general anaesthesia in this age
group.

REFERENCES

1. Berkowitz S, Green B.A. 1951. Spinal anesthesia in
   children: Report based on 350 patients under 13 years of
   age. Anesthesiology, 12:376
2. Campbell M.F. 1933. Caudal anesthesia in children. J.
   Urol. 30:245
3. Eriksson E. 1965. Axillary brachial plexus anaesthesia in
   children with citanest. Acta Anaesthesiol. Scand. 16:291
4. Farr R.E. 1920. Local anesthesia in infancy and
   childhood. Arch. Pediatr. 37:381

5. Fortin G, Tremblay L. 1959. The short-needle technique in brachial plexus block. Can. Anaesth. Soc. J. 6:32

6. Gouveia M.A. 1970. Raquianesthesia para pacientes pediatricos Rev.Bras.Anest. 4:503

7. Gray T. 1910. Study of spinal anaesthesia in infants and children. Lancet 10:10 1909; and 10:6

8. Isakob Y.F., Geraskin B.I., Koshevnikov V.A. 1971. Long term peridural anesthesia after operations on the organs of the chest in children. Grudnaja Chirurija 13:104

9. Niesel H.C., Rodrigues P, Wilsmann I. 1974. Regionalanaesthesie der oberen Extremität bei Kindern. Anaesthesist 32:178

10. Schulte-Steinberg O., Rahlfs V.W. 1977. Spread of extradural analgesia following caudal injection in children: A statistical study. Brit. J. Anaesth. 49:1027

11. Schulte-Steinberg O., in Wüst H.J., Schulte-Steinberg O. 1983 in press. Epiduralanaesthesie bei Kindern und älteren Patienten Springer-Verlag Berlin Heidelberg New York Tokyo

12. Sievers R. 1936. Peridural Anaesthesie zur Cystoscopie beim Kind. Arch. Klin. Chir. 185:395

13. Winnie A.P. 1970 Interscalene brachial plexus block. Anesth. Analg. (Cleve) 49:455

CELIAC PLEXUS BLOCK

Daniel C. Moore

INTRODUCTION

In 1919 Kappis [1] described percutaneous celiac plexus block. Since then, variations and refinements in his technique have been proposed, including the use of roentgenographic techniques to improve results and to avoid complications, particularly when neurolytic drugs are injected for relief of intractable cancer pain [2-6].

The purpose of this review of celiac plexus block is to capsulize our knowledge of this technique through 1983, which has been made possible by modern roentgenography, particularly CT (computerized tomography).

INDICATIONS

Celiac plexus block may be used to complement bilateral block of the lower seven intercostal nerves for intra-abdominal surgery by eliminating visceral pain transmitted by nerve fibers which accompany the vagus and the splanchnic nerves. However, its principle uses are: (1) the differentiation of visceral from somatic pain; (2) the location of visceral pain, that is upper or lower abdomen; and (3) the alleviation of intractable pain from cancer that is limited to one or more of the following upper intra-abdominal organs: (a) stomach and/or duodenum, (b) liver, (c) gallbladder, (d) pancreas, and (e) adrenal glands. Its most frequent use is to alleviate pain from cancer of the pancreas.

Seldom does celiac plexus block with either a local anesthetic drug or a neurolytic drug provide prolonged pain relief of acute or chronic pancreatitis. On the other hand, local anesthetic solutions containing steroids (80 mg of methylprednisolone

[Depo-Medrol®] or triamcinolone [Aristocort®] in 50 ml of 0.5% bupivacaine (250 mg) with epinephrine 1:200,000 [0.25 mg in 50 ml]) have produced some promising results in treating acute pancreatitis with celiac plexus block, provided that one or more blocks are done early in the course of the disease.

ANATOMY

To perform a successful celiac plexus block and avoid complications the following anatomy of the nerves which form the celiac plexus and its ganglia and their relationship to the kidneys and diaphragm must be understood [7].

Celiac Plexus and Ganglia: The greater (T5-8 or 9), lesser (T9, 10, 11), and lowest (from the last thoracic ganglion) splanchnic nerves of both sides and some filaments from the vagus nerves, mainly the right, pass through the prevertebral space of the thorax, pierce the diaphragm, and form the celiac plexus and ganglia (Figure 1).

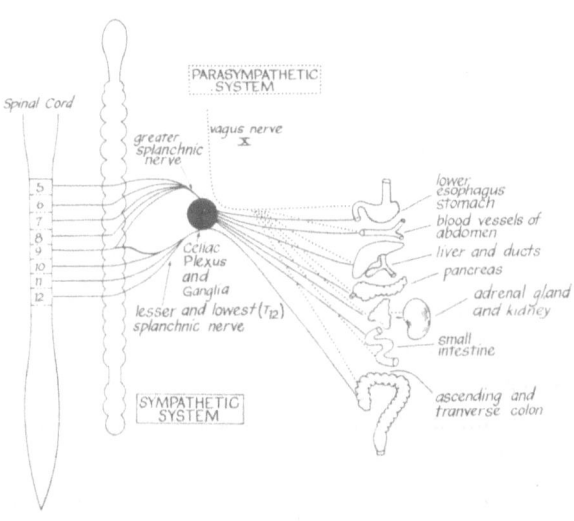

Figure 1. Schematic drawing of the components of the celiac plexus and ganglia.

The plexus gives off secondary plexuses to the diaphragm, liver, spleen, stomach, suprarenal gland, kidney, spermatic cord, abdominal aorta, and mesentery. The plexus is situated at the level of the upper part of the first lumbar vertebra and is composed of a right and left celiac ganglion and a dense network of nerve fibers connecting them. It surrounds the celiac artery and the base of the superior mesenteric artery. It lies in areolar tissue behind the peritoneum, the stomach, and the omental bursa; just caudad to (below and in front of) the crura of the diaphragm and the commencement of the abdominal aorta; and between the suprarenal glands.

Kidneys: It is important to remember that the kidneys: (1) lie adjacent to the vertebral column and behind the peritoneum, (2) extend from above the body of the twelfth thoracic vertebra to below the second lumbar vertebra (Figure 2A), and (3) are surrounded by loose areolar tissue and a mass of fat. They are in the same compartment with the celiac plexus, the aorta, and the vena cava. Moreover, the medial surfaces of the upper poles of the kidneys lie approximately 5 cm (2 inches) and their lower poles 7 cm (3 inches), from the midline of the back (the spinous processes of the vertebrae) with the right kidney 1.3 cm (1/2 inch) lower than the left (Figure 2B). Also, the upper poles are at the level of the twelfth thoracic vertebra and the lower poles at the upper border of the body of the third lumbar vertebra (Figure 2A,B). Finally, the twelfth ribs lie over the kidneys (Figure 2B).

Therefore, if puncture of the kidneys is to be avoided, the needles must pass medial to them in the 2 to 3 cm (3/4 to 1-1/4 inches) of tissue which normally lies between the kidneys and the lumbar vertebra [2,3]. In the patient with cancer, this distance may be markedly reduced on one or both sides by pressure from the tumor (Figure 10) [3].

Diaphragm: The right crus of the diaphragm, broader and longer than the left, arises from the anterolateral surfaces of the bodies of the upper three lumbar vertebrae and from their intervertebral discs, while the left crus arises from the corresponding parts of the upper two.

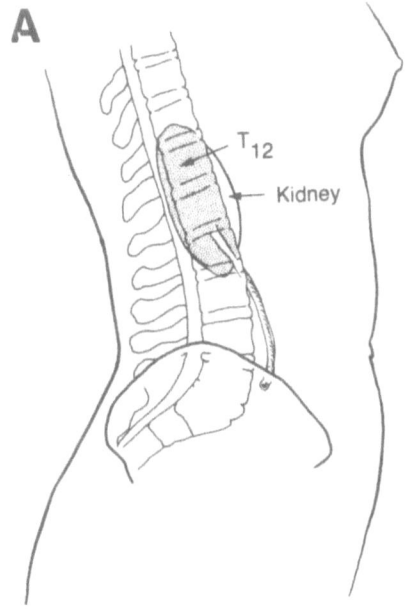

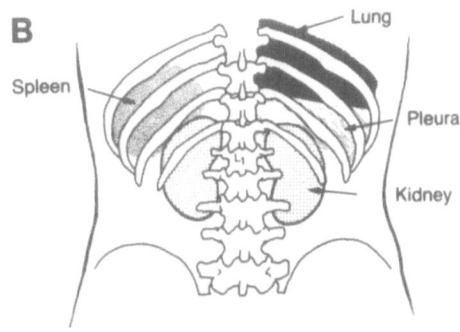

Figure 2. A. Schematic drawing showing position of kidneys lateral and opposite to vertebral column. B. Schematic drawing of back of lumbar region, showing position of kidneys in relationship to vertebrae, twelfth rib, pleura, lungs, and spleen.

TECHNICAL CONSIDERATIONS

Celiac plexus block is not difficult to master, and complications are minimal provided the technique of the block is meticulously followed [2,6].

Approaches: The celiac plexus may be blocked in one of three ways: (1) the classic approach, that is, placing the needles and the solution cephalad to (above) the diaphragm and blocking the greater, lesser, and lowest splanchnic as well as the vagus nerves, that is, the nerves which form the celiac plexus; (2) the transcrural approach, which results in blocking the celiac plexus and its ganglia caudad to (below) the diaphragm; or (3) a combination of these.

Since 1919 [1] and regardless of the drug to be injected, the classic approach is the one most frequently used for diagnostic and therapeutic blocks without the aid of roentgenographic techniques. If the transcrural approach is to be employed, CT is essential for accurate needle placement. Whether the transcrural approach has any advantage over the classic approach for the initial attempt to relieve the pain of cancer with a neurolytic drug is debatable [5].

Position (Figure 3): For any of the approaches, the patient is placed in the prone position with a pillow between the iliac crests and the rib cage so as to reduce the lumbar curve of the vertebral column to a minimum. Any other position increases significantly the likelihood of misplacing the needles.

Landmarks (Figure 3): The landmarks are the spinous process of the first lumbar vertebra and its cephalad edge under which the celiac plexus lies, and the lower borders of the twelfth ribs a maximum of 7.5 cm (3 inches) from the posterior midline of the body. These points are marked with Xs, and the Xs are connected by straight lines forming a flat triangle. The maximum of 7.5 cm from the midline to the ribs is critical because of the anatomical position of the kidneys (Figure 2B). If puncture of the kidneys is to be avoided, the needles must pass medial to them in the 2 to 3 cm (1 inch) of tissue which lies between the medial edges of the kidneys and the lumbar vertebrae. When the distance for inserting the needle is greater than 7.5 cm from the midline, the needle is more likely to pass through the kidney [3].

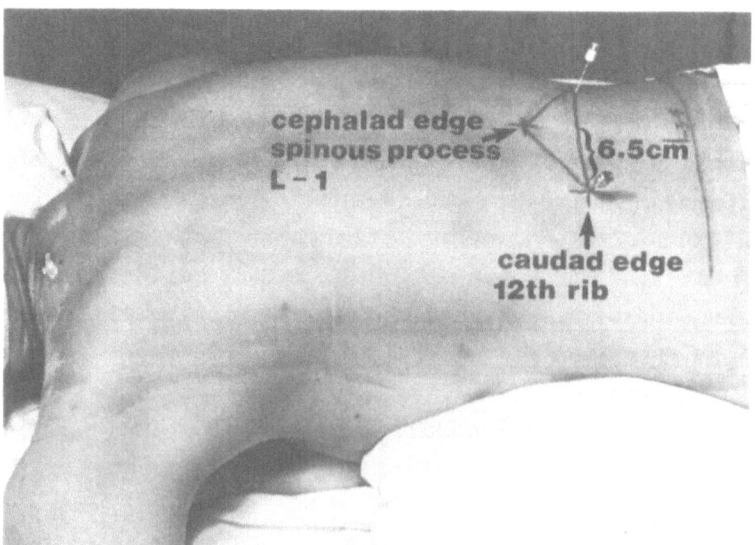

Figure 3. Position, landmarks, and needles in place for the classic approach for celiac plexus block.

Classic Approach (Needle's Bevels Placed Cephalad to the Diaphragm) (Figure 4, 5, 6A): A 20-gauge needle is placed through the X at the lower edge of the twelfth rib, at a 45° angle to the skin, on the left side. With the line of the side of the marked triangle as a guide, the needle is slowly advanced until its point contacts the lateral surface of the body of the first lumbar vertebra. The depth of the needle is noted. Then the needle is withdrawn 2.5 cm (1 inch), and the angle between its shaft and the skin is increased by approximately 10°--that is, from 45° to 60°-- and then the needle is reinserted. This maneuver is repeated, increasing the angle slightly each time, until the needle is felt to slip off the body of the vertebra. Then it is inserted to a depth of 2 to 2.5 cm deeper than when the first contact with the lateral surface of the vertebra was made or until pulsations of the aorta are felt. If pulsations are felt, then the needle is withdrawn 3 to 4 mm (1/8 to 3/16 inch) so as to be certain it does not lie in the wall of the aorta (Figure 6). After placement of this needle, another 20-gauge needle is placed on the right side in an identical way and to the same or a slightly deeper depth as the needle on the left side.

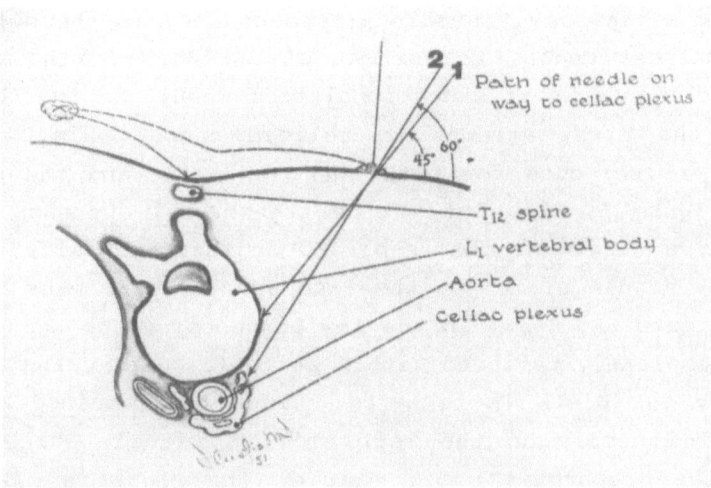

Figure 4. Schematic drawing of method of needle placement. Needle 1, initial insertion. Needle 2, walked off body of first lumbar vertebra.

48

Transcrural Approach (Needle's Bevel Caudad to the Diaphragm) (Figure 7A): All the steps of the classic approach are followed except one needle only is placed on the right side and advanced 4 to 5 cm (1 3/4 to 2 inches) or more anterior to the body of the vertebra so that its bevel traverses the right crus of the diaphragm.

Combined Approach (Figure 8): The needle on the left is placed as described for the classic approach (Figure 5, 6A) and the needle on the right as for the transcrural approach (Figure 7A, 8A).

ROENTGENOGRAPHIC CONSIDERATIONS

Other than cost which may be considered a disadvantage of the use of roentgenography, the following are the advantages and dis-advantages of employing them as aids.

Indications: When performing a diagnostic and/or a thera-peutic block today, I prefer to employ a combination of the avail-able roentgenographic techniques, namely, posteroanterior and lateral roentgenograms when doing a diagnostic block with the local anesthetic drug (Figure 5, 9) and CT when executing a thera-peutic block with alcohol (Figure 6, 7, 8, 10) [3]. Doing so gives documentation of needle placement and, if the solution con-tains contrast media, the extent of spread. Furthermore, using these techniques is an educational tool when teaching residents.

For the first attempt to relieve cancer pain, the classic approach is selected for both the diagnostic and the therapeutic block (Figure 5, 6). But if the transcrural approach is chosen, then only a single needle is placed on the right side (Figure 7A) because a needle placed on the left usually will pass through the aorta (Figure 6A, 8A). In the few instances where the cancer pain is not completely relieved within 24 to 48 hours using the classic approach, the block is repeated. Then the combined approach is used. The needle on the left side is placed behind the aorta (above the diaphragm) while that on the right is placed trans-crurally (below it) (Figure 8A).

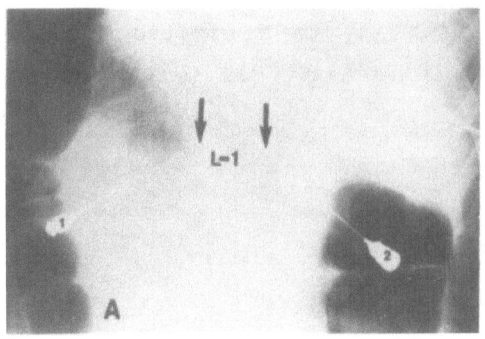 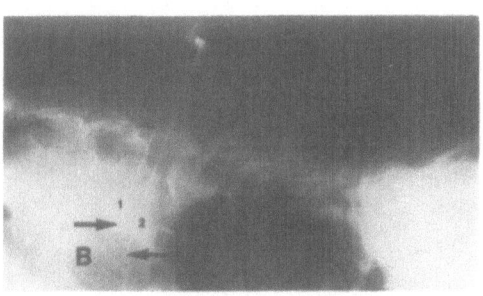

Figure 5. Classic Approach. (A) Posteroanterior
roentgenogram of needles depicted in most publications to be correctly and optimally placed for celiac
plexus block anterior to and at cephalad lateral borders of body of first lumbar vertebra. These needles
were placed by contacting the body of the first lumbar vertebra, walking the needles off the body of the
vertebra and then advancing them inward 1.5 to 2 cm
[6]. (B) Lateral view of A shows needle on left and
right anterior to body of vertebra. Although both
needles are the same depth, the right one appears,
from distortion, to be deeper than the left. Note
that the needle on the right contains a removable
metal cap so that it may be differentiated from the
left on the lateral roentgenogram.

Needle Placement: A posteroanterior roentgenogram can help
avoid misplacement of the needles if: (a) there is a congenital
absence of the twelfth rib or if it is short and not palpable
(this occurs in approximately 20% of patients); (b) the twelfth
rib slopes markedly caudad; or (c) six lumbar vertebrae are present (Figure 9) [3]. With CT, such variations cannot be
demonstrated as rapidly. A lateral roentgenogram can assure that
the needle does not traverse an intervertebral foramen and that
the needle's point is positioned anterior to the body of the first
lumbar vertebra (Figure 5B) [3].

On the other hand, posteroanterior and lateral roentgenograms
are of no value in establishing whether the needle has punctured
an organ, the exact distance its point is located anterior to the
first lumbar vertebra, or the exact spread of the injected solution (Figure 5A,B) [3]. Fluoroscopy has the same advantages and

drawbacks as roentgenography, but with it, to a limited extent, the spread of a radiopaque solution in relationship to the pulsations of the aorta can be followed.

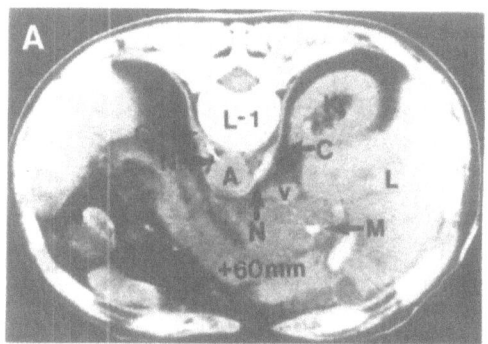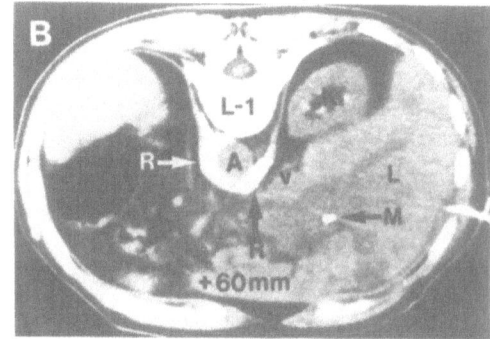

Figure 6. (A) CT at +60 mm (6 cm) cephalad from start of scanning (hubs of needles), with bevel of needle on left positioned unintentionally in wall of aorta and needle on right in correct position. (B) CT at +60 mm, needle on left was withdrawn approximately 3 mm to free it from wall of aorta. Then 50 ml of 50% alcohol containing megulmine iothalamate was injected, that is, 25 ml through each needle, and both needles were withdrawn. The solution spread cephalad to the diaphragm and surrounded the aorta. L-1 = first lumbar vertebra. A = aorta. v = vena cava. M and arrow = drainage tube in bile duct. C and arrows - crura of diaphragm. K = kidney. L = liver. Ns and arrows = points of needles. R and arrows = alcohol-iothalamate - local anesthetic drug solution.

CT confirms the topographic anatomy of the kidney and further demonstrates that in order to avoid puncture of the kidneys in all patients, the site of insertion of the needles must be no more than 7 to 7.5 cm from the spinous process of the lumbar vertebra directly medial to the lower edge of the twelfth rib (Figures 6-8) [3]. Even this distance may be too great in a patient with a large tumor because a needle has passed through the kidney when these distances were not exceeded (Figure 10) [3].

When the needle is to be placed caudad to the diaphragm, CT is mandatory to be sure that the needle has traversed the diaphragm and lies below it (Figure 7A, 8B).

Spread of Solution: If during the diagnostic block, the anesthetic solution contains a radiopaque material the extent of its spread can only be only be estimated.   Therefore, seldom is such a material added.

On the other hand, with CT the injected solution always contains a radiopaque material which permits accurate tracking of the areas through which it spreads in relationship to the organs (Figures 6B, 7B, 8C). This is particularly helpful if one or both blocks fail to relieve the patient's pain.   Furthermore and contrary to another study [4,5], it should be noted that when the transcrural approach is used, the solution does not spread around the aorta, as it does with the classic approach (compare Figure 6B with Figure 7B and 8C).

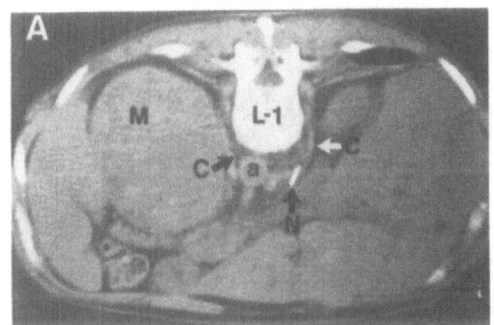 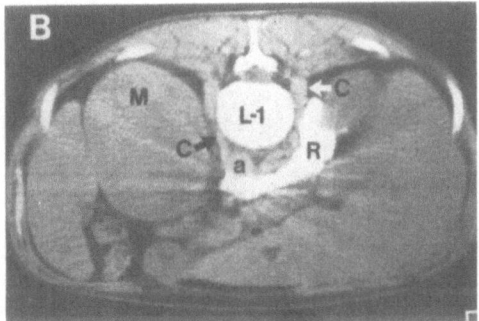

Figure 7. When the transcrural approach is employed, usually only one needle is placed on the right side at L1 because, even if CT is used, a needle inserted on the left side would in most instances pass through the aorta prior to puncturing the crus of the diaphragm, as can be ascertained from the CT scan. (A) Needle's bevel anterior to crus of diaphragm. (B) Spread from needle in A of 50 ml of 50% alcohol containing meglumine iothalamate. L1 = body of first lumbar vertebra. C = crura of diaphragm. a = aorta. M = massive growth of lung metastasis in left adrenal gland. N = needle's bevel. R = spread of radiopaque solution in prevertebral space anterior to (below) diaphragm.

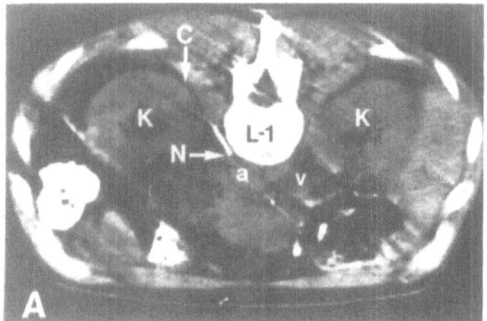
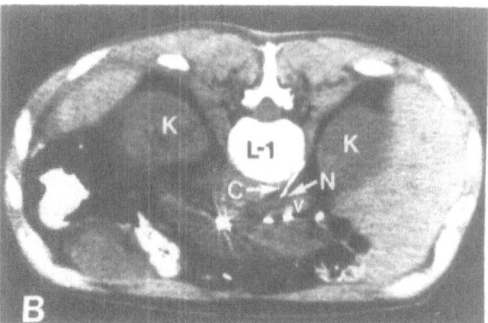
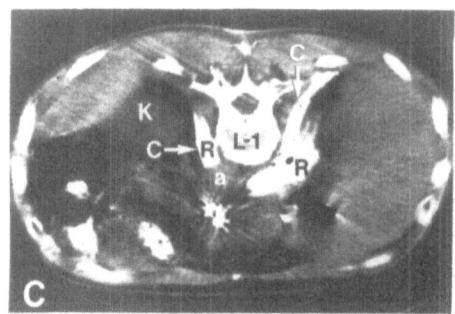

Figure 8. CT of a combined approach in a patient whose previous block using classic approach gave only partial relief. A. Needle on left cephalad to (above) diaphragm. B. Needle on right caudad to (below) diaphragm. C. Spread of solution following injection of 30 ml of 50% alcohol containing meglumine iothalamate through needle on left and 50 ml through needle on right. L-1 = 1st lumbar vertebra. K = kidneys. C = crus of diaphragm. N = needle's point. a = aorta. v = vena cava. R = spread of radiopaque solution.

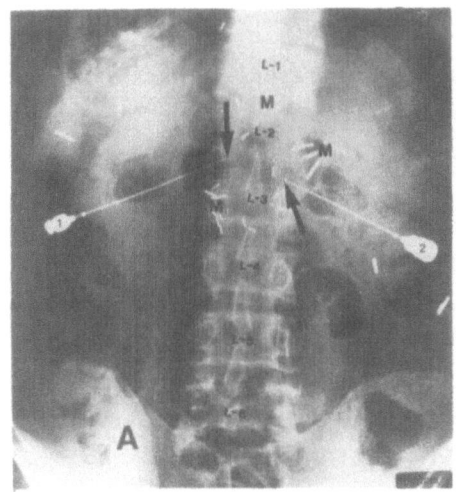 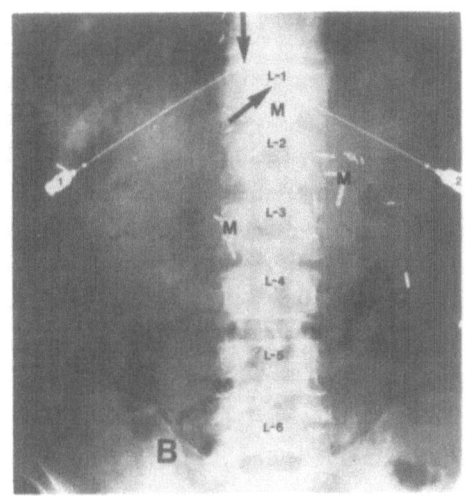

Figure 9. A. Initial insertion of needle resulted in misplacement at second lumbar vertebra because patient has six lumbar vertebrae and marked slope of 12th rib. B. Needles adjusted to correct position at L-1.

DRUG CONSIDERATIONS

Diagnostic Block: The classic approach is routinely used for a diagnostic block (Figures 5, 6). And, 50 ml of 0.5% bupivacaine (250 mg) with 1:200,000 epinephrine is injected, that is, 25 ml through each needle at the rate of 1.0 ml/second.

Therapeutic Block: Using either the classic or the one needle transcrural approach, 50 ml of solution is injected which contains: (1) 25 ml absolute alcohol, (2) 7 ml of meglumine iothalamate USP 60 (600 mg/ml), osmolarity = 1.5 mOsm/ml (Conray® 60%) and (3) 18 ml of 0.75% bupivacaine. This solution also is injected at the rate of 1 ml/second (Figure 6B, 7B).

On the other hand, when the initial block does not relieve the cancer pain, the block is repeated employing the combined approach. 80 ml of solution is injected which contains: (1) 40 ml absolute alcohol, (2) 8 ml of the meglumine iothalamate, and (3) 32 ml of 0.75% bupivacaine. Then 30 ml is injected through the needle behind the aorta and 50 ml through the other one (Figure 8B)

COMPLICATIONS

If the needles are placed correctly as described, that is, no more than 7.5 cm from the spinous process of the lumbar vertebra, immediately below the caudad edge of the twelfth rib and anterior to the body of the first lumbar vertebra, either cephalad to or caudad to the diaphragm and verified by conventional roentgenography and/or CT, the only complication which should occur is hypotension, primarily orthostatic, for 24 hours [6]. Therefore, intravenous fluids should be running during and following the block. And, if the patient is to ambulate, orders must be specific to prevent the patient fainting (elastic stockings, a tight abdominal binder, etc.) and falling (assistance when walking) [6]. Also, back pain lasting 24 to 36 hours may result from the alcohol. The intractable cancer pain usually disappears within 15 minutes, but occasionally it persists, even though markedly less intense, for 24 hours.

On the other hand, if the needles are incorrectly inserted through the skin more than 7.5 cm from the spinous process of a lumbar vertebra and if placement is not verified by posteroanterior roentgenograms or CT, one or more of the following complications may develop: (1) the kidney may be impaled (Figure 10), with subsequent hematuria, and if the pelvis of the kidney is also punctured, urine may extravasate into the tissues; (2) a lumbar somatic nerve may be blocked, with a motor and sensory deficit in the lower extremity; (3) the needle(s) may pass into the epidural or subarachnoid space, which, if not recognized, will result in epidural or spinal block; or (4) the lung(s) may be punctured and pneumothorax may result.

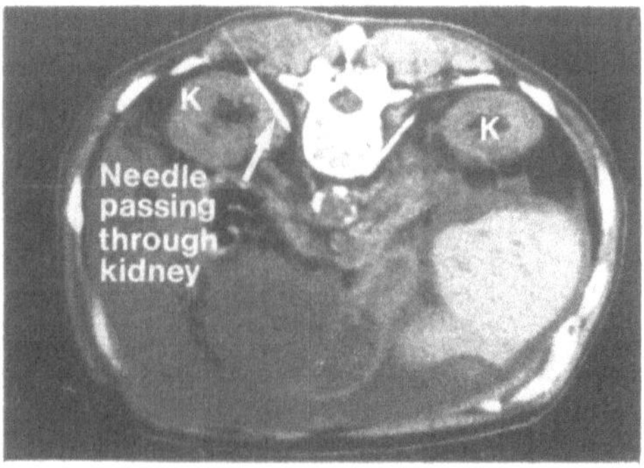

Figure 10. Needle inserted 6 cm (2 1/4 inch) from spine of vertebra, passing through cortex of left kidney which lies closer to body of vertebra from pressure of tumor. Note distance of right kidney from body of vertebra is greater than usual. K = kidney.

Obviously, if these occur with a diagnostic block using a local anesthetic solution and if they are recognized and properly treated, permanent sequelae are unlikely to result. On the other hand, if a neurolytic therapeutic block is executed, the patient may be permanently paralyzed or lose the kidney. Both of these things have happened.

In conclusion, to avoid the complications of celiac plexus block, it is mandatory that the twelfth rib and the first lumbar vertebra be identified, and that the distance from the midline to the point of needle insertion not exceed 7.5 cm. Furthermore, roentgenography can assure correct needle placement and avoid complications.

REFERENCES

1. Kappis M: Sensibilitat und lokale anasthesie im chirurgischen gebeit der bauchkokle mit besonderer berucksichtigung der splanchnicusanasthesie. Beitr Klin Chir 1919;115:161-75.
2. Moore DC: Celiac (splanchnic) plexus block with alcohol for cancer pain of the upper intra-abdominal viscera. Advances in Pain Research and Therapy. Bonica JJ, Ventafrida V. (eds) 1979;2:357-71.
3. Moore DC, Bush WH, Burnett LL: Celiac plexus blocks; a roentgenographic, anatomic study of technique and spread of solution in patients and corpses. Anesth Analg 1981;60:369-79.
4. Singler RC: An improved technique for alcohol neurolysis of the celiac plexus. Anesthesiology 1982;56:137-41.
5. Moore DC, Bush WH, Burnett LL/Singler RC: An improved technique for celiac plexus block may be more theoretical than real (correspondence). Anesthesiology 1982;57:347-9.
6. Moore DC: Regional Block. 4th ed. Springfield, IL. Charles C Thomas, 1965;148,149-56,156-8,332-3.
7. Gray H: Anatomy of the Human Body. 36th ed. Williams PL, Warwick R, ed.Philadelphia: Lea and Febiger, 1980;549,1131, 1387.

SYMPATHETIC DYSTROPHIES: I.V. REGIONAL GUANETHIDINE VERSUS
STELLATE GANGLION BLOCKS

JOHN G. HANNINGTON-KIFF

Introduction

The established method of temporarily blocking the sympathetic nerve supply to the upper extremity is injection of
the stellate ganglion with local anaesthetic solution. Though
disliked by the average patient, because it involves penetration of the neck, the stellate ganglion block has the advantage of being quickly performed by the expert. The principal
disadvantage arises from the associated sympathetic block
which occurs in the face. In fact unwanted facial effects are
normally used as an indication of successful stellate ganglion block. It is possible to minimise the facial sympathetic blockade by attention to technique with the patient
sitting upright to encourage the local anaesthetic to flow to
lower levels of the cervical chain but the outcome is unpredictable. More serious is the occasional pneumothorax which
occurs, though this is usually the result of poor technique
or the use of the less popular posterior paravertebral approach to the region of the stellate ganglion. A frequent
nuisance is the hoarse voice caused by anaesthesia of the
recurrent laryngeal nerve.

Another disadvantage is the short duration of the block
which will be commensurate with the period of activity of the
local anaesthetic agent used. Attempts to procure prolonged
interruption of the sympathetic supply by the use of neurolytic agents should be reserved for the seriously ill patient
because of the persistence of unwanted effects in the face
and larynx and the possibility of hazardous complications.
The common state of affairs is that patients require a series
of stellate ganglion blocks if anything more than a diagnostic test is desired. Many patients refuse to complete a
prescribed course of stellate ganglion blocks because they
run out of courage.

My interest in the rehabilitation of hands, especially
those affected by various kinds of sympathetic dystrophy, led
me to look for an alternative method of blocking the sympathetic nerve supply in the upper extremity. It occurred to me
to try attacking the sympathetic nerve endings by injecting a
noradrenergic neuron blocking drug into the peripheral veins
of a limb isolated by an arterial tourniquet in a kind of
Bier block. I found guanethidine ideal for this purpose and
the results obtained have transformed my success-rate in the
relief of sympathetic dystrophies affecting limbs compared
with my former experience with sympathetic ganglion blocks.

At a stroke I had also found a solution to two clinical problems. One was the provision of sympathetic blockade in a limb to which sympathetic tone had returned after surgical sympathectomy. The other problem was providing sympathetic blockade in patients who were on continuous anticoagulant therapy. In the first instance, a "stellate ganglion block" would be to no avail after surgical excision of the stellate ganglion. In the second instance serious uncontrollable haemorrhage could occur after deep penetration of tissues by an injection in a patient with impaired clotting mechanisms. Apart from the general effects of the loss of blood, the local pressure caused by a collection of blood could adversely affect the base of the neck and pleura. Finally, the use of guanethidine blocks has given rise to many new ideas about the aetiology of certain enigmatic painful disabilities affecting the limbs.

Principle of guanethidine blockade

In the intravenous regional (IVR) technique, a high concentration of a drug such as guanethidine can be achieved in the tissues of the limb whilst avoiding systemic effects. In this kind of "pharmacological target block" guanethidine is selectively taken up by noradrenergic nerve endings. Guanethidine has a high affinity for its target and there is a tendency for guanethidine to be progressively accumulated by noradrenergic neurons. The first effect of the guanethidine is to release noradrenaline (NA) from its storage sites in the postganglionic nerve endings. This fact must be taken into consideration in the clinical use of guanethidine in the IVR technique and this will be discussed in a subsequent section. It is important to realise that the sympathetic nervous system (unlike a cholinergic effector system) relies upon recapturing its transmitter, in this case NA, from the synaptic cleft. Guanethidine inhibits this reuptake of NA and in prolonged or high concentration guanethidine can permanently damage the neuronal "reuptake pump" for NA. In high concentration (e.g. over 30 mg/kg) guanethidine can actually cause the noradrenergic nerve endings to retract from their effector sites. The increased gap in the synaptic cleft produces in effect a microsurgical terminal sympathectomy.

It is notable that guanthidine produces a pure noradrenergic neuron block unlike a sympathetic ganglion block with local anaesthetic which will interrupt any cholinergic efferents and any sensory fibres in the vicinity. I have found that an ice challenge-test elsewhere in the body (e.g. the opposite hand) causes a paradoxical vasodilatation in the limb treated with guanethidine instead of the vasoconstriction normally encountered. This is indirect evidence in favour of the existence of cholinergic vasodilator fibres which are refuted by many physiologists. The fact that a guanethidine block which is wholly the result of efferent blockade can arrest the pain in causalgia, for example, is the first incontrovertible proof that such a condition is not subserved by afferent fibres travelling in the sympathetic nervous system. Though guanethidine is said by some to have mild local anaesthetic properties, I have never been able to demonstrate this clinically, and the effect referred to is probably the result of a weak membrane stabilising effect which reduces the action potential.

The guanethidine technique

The solution for injection is prepared by drawing up the guanethidine into a 50 ml syringe and then aspirating saline until the desired volume is reached in the syringe. The dose of guanethidine is 10-30 mg and an average dilution-volume for the arm is 30 ml total. The precise quantities should be varied according to the size of the limb, the fitness and age of the patient and whether it is a diagnostic, initial or repeated therapeutic block. The tourniquet time is 20 minutes. The tourniquet can be deflated as soon as 7 minutes but some side effects such as a slight dry, burning sensation in the throat may be experienced by the patient. I have never experienced serious side effects when the tourniquet is released and I have never had to reinflate the tourniquet. I release the tourniquet in one step as a routine. I favour giving patients a light general anaesthetic following intravenous induction and maintenance with nitrous oxide and oxygen. However, patients without a painful limb in the first instance are on the whole able to withstand the relative discomfort of the tourniquet and do not need general anaesthesia.

A smaller dose of guanethidine, say 10 mg, should be used in diagnostic blocks when an early vasodilatation is desired. It has been mentioned that the first effect of guanethidine is to release NA. This causes a delay in vasodilatation and, indeed, when a bigger dose of guanethidine is given as a first dose the full vasodilatation and therefore increase in warmth may not be evident for some hours. The inexperienced operator may think that the block has not worked in these circumstances if he only observes the patient for a short time. The patient should be warned that the limb might be warmest on the following day and not to think that he has developed an infection in the arm.

At a subsequent block carried out within a few days a higher dose of guanethidine can be given with less likelihood of releasing NA because the neuron will have been "self-tamed" by the guanethidine lingering in the neuron. Guanethidine can remain to some degree within the neuron for up to 21 days.

There is a word of caution: patients with a history of Raynaud's phenomenon are very sensitive to NA and should be given a reduced dose of guanethidine, certainly at the first treatment. They will not come to systemic harm but the limb will show marked pilo-erection (a specific effect of NA in any patient) and the onset of vasodilatation will be delayed. Another way of approaching these patients and if wished any other patients for an initial block is to precede the guanethidine (by about one or two minutes after inflation of the tourniquet) by an injection of a small dose of an alpha-adrenoceptor blocking drug such as thymoxamine. This will block the effect of the NA flushed out by the guanethidine.

The initial release of NA by the guanethidine block is probably the reason for the initial brief period of burning in limbs affected by causalgia and related types of sympathetic dysaesthesia. This can be a useful diagnostic test in some puzzling limb pains. This burning pain can be alleviated or avoided in the conscious patient by adding a small quantity of local anaesthetic to the guanethidine solution. An alpha-adrenoceptor blocking agent will also protect the patient from an exacerbation of pain triggered by the NA. But it should be borne in mind that the alpha adrenoceptor blocker will interfere slightly with the entry of guanethidine into the neuron and slightly reduce the eventual potency of the block.

Indications for guanethidine blocks

Pain and disability

The type of pain which responds to guanethidine block is that associated with hyperpathia and sensitivity to cold. Interestingly, these two associated findings also disappear after guanethidine block. This, however, is not specific to guanethidine block but also occurs after sympathetic ganglion block.

It is surprising how guanethidine blocks can relieve stiffness and guarding in the muscles of limbs, especially the small muscles of the hands, in reflex sympathetic dystrophy syndromes (algodystrophy syndromes). I believe that this is the result of the removal of excessive sympathetic drive to the muscle spindles and is not simply the effect of alleviating pain. Guanethidine blocks have also produced quite dramatic relief of "thalamic" limb pain associated with cerebro-vascular accidents. This finding merits further study.

Vascular disorders

Guanethidine blockade has solved the problem of what to do for patients who have deteriorating circulation or the resumption of pain associated with the return of sympathetic tone after previously adequate surgical sympathectomy. This return of sympathetic tone is not uncommon within a year or so of surgical sympathectomy.

In the case of vasospastic disorders such as Raynaud's phenomenon in which there is sensitivity to cold, a patient can be tided over the winter months with perhaps 2 or 3 guanethidine blocks. Bearing in mind that surgical sympathectomy is not reliably permanent, this is a very useful therapeutic approach.

It is worth noting that guanethidine blocks are anti-NA and are therefore inappropriate in the treatment of excessive sweating in the extremities. It will be recalled that sweating has a cholinergic mechanism. A corollary of this is that a guanethidine-blocked hand remains moist which is necessary for a good grip. This is an important point in hand rehabili-

60

tation.

Osteodystropy

Bone scans have shown that the high turnover osteoporosis
in the active stage of Sudeck's atrophy can be halted in a
remarkable way by even one guanethidine block. I have had the
opportunity of studying a series of patients with the rare
disorder of regional migratory osteolysis who over a period
of months or years have required treatment of painful episodes of osteoporosis in successive limbs. On each occasion
guanethidine blocks have been effective and I wonder whether
it is justifiable to conclude that the trigger to this regional osteolysis is NA. Perhaps there is a cascade of events
involving prostaglandin, which substance is known to cause
osteoporosis, and I am working upon this hypothesis with the
aid of antiprostaglandin blocks using a parenteral form of
aspirin. There is, of course, an opportunity to employ a
variety of drugs successively in the intravenous regional
technique in an effort to identify possible chemical triggers
of painful limb disorders and to provide rational therapy
upon this basis.

Guide to further reading

1. Hannington-Kiff J.G. 1980. In Limbo. Jacksonian Prize
   Dissertation, in libris, Royal College of Surgeons of
   England.
2. Hannington-Kiff J.G. 1982. Hyperadrenergic-effected limb
   causalgia: relief by i.v. pharmacologic norepinephrine
   blockade. American Heart Journal 103: 152-153.
3. Hannington-Kiff J.G. Antisympathetic drugs in limbs. In:
   Textbook of Pain, edited by Melzack R and Wall P.D. (in
   press).

SURFACE LANDMARKS FOR SUPRACLAVICULAR BRACHIAL PLEXUS BLOCK.

L.J. DUPRE, P. STIEGLITZ.

Brachial plexus block is an alternative to general anesthesia frequently used for surgery on the upper extremities, particularly in emergency operations. Techniques for blocking the plexus involve infiltration at one of four blocking areas : paravertebral, supraclavicular, infraclavicular or in the axilla. The supraclavicular approach has several advantages : the brachial plexus is blocked where it is most compactly arranged ; all the branches can be anesthetized through one single injection and with small amount of solution. The technique can be performed with the arm in virtually any position (1). Some drawbacks cannot be neglected. There is a risk of pneumothorax, even if the incidence of such a complication is very small (less than 0,5 %) (2). Furthermore, considerable experience is required to master a technique (3) which is rather difficult to describe and teach (1).

Kulenkampff, the first to describe the supraclavicular approach (4) insisted on the structures limiting the working field : "the clavicle marking the lower limit, the first rib the upper, and the subclavian artery the outer limit of safety". Since this description, many improvements have been suggested (5, 6, 7, 8, 9, 10). They all aim to facilitate the location of the subclavian artery which is the surest guide to the brachial plexus (1). But whatever the technique, the subclavian artery pulse may not be felt if the clavicle is raised, if the platysma muscle is tense, or if the patient is obese. The first rib provides good protection against accidental pleural puncture. However, locating the arterial pulse by pressing the finger into the supraclavicular fossa, as recommanded by Kulenkampff and Persky is frequently illusory. Interpretation of the classical "downward, backward, and inward direction" for insertion of the needle may be inappropriate, and not always prevent the penetration of the pleura. For these reasons, particularly for the anesthesiologist who has had little opportunity during his training to develop expertise with supraclavicular brachial plexus block, the risk of failure and/or pneumothorax is an important deterrent.

Therefore, we have attempted to develop a technique based on readily recognized surface landmarks (10, 11).

ANATOMIC CONSIDERATIONS

The brachial plexus is formed from the anterior primary rami of the fifth, sixth, seventh and eighth cervical and first thoracic spinal nerves, with occasional twigs from the fourth cervical and the second thoracic nerves. The roots emerge between the anterior and middle scalene muscles to unite and form three trunks. These trunks converge towards the upper side of the first rib where they are arranged one above the other, vertically according to their designation (superior, middle, inferior). As these branches pass downward and laterally behind the clavicle, to enter the axilla, they are assembled into cords (lateral, medial and posterior) which divide into the great nerves of the upper extremities.

The supraclavicular fossa or posterior cervical triangle of the neck (13) consists of the area enclosed by the posterior margin of the sternocleidomastoïd muscle, the middle third of the clavicle, and the anterior edge of the trapezius muscle. The brachial plexus lies superior and posterior to the subclavian artery, which is located at the floor of the posterior cervical triangle.

Other anatomic findings can be reported in addition to the classical relationships of the plexus in the supraclavicular fossa. Thus, a line drawn between the internal clavicular insertion of trapezius muscle and the top of supraclavicularis minor fossa (14) (the triangle formed by the clavicular and sternal heads of the sternocleidomastoïd muscle and the clavicle) crosses the external jugular vein just above the brachial plexus (fig.1). In fact, the plexus lies under the skin, slightly lateral to the perpendicular projection of the crossing point, at a depth of 1 to 2,5 cm.

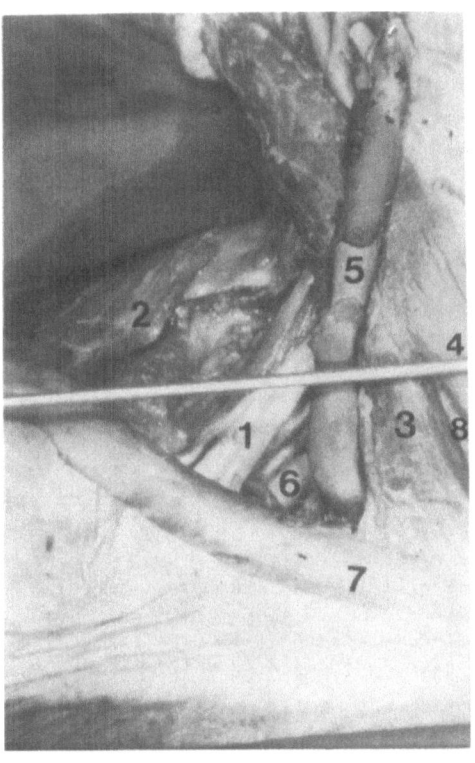

Fig. 1. Anatomy.

1 = brachial plexus
2 = trapezius muscle
3 = clavicular head
4 = sternal head (3 and 4
  comprise the sternocleidomastoïd muscle)
5 = external jugular vein
6 = subclavian artery
7 = clavicle
8 = fossa supraclavicularis
  minor

The anatomic considerations suggest that brachial plexus block by supraclavicular approach can be performed using such surface landmarks as the external jugular vein, the clavicular insertion of the trapezius muscle and the sternocleidomastoïd muscle.

TECHNIQUE

Position and landmarks : the patient should lie in the dorsal recumbent position, arms at the side, the head on a small pillow and turned away from the side to be anesthezized. The patient is then instructed to raise his head, putting strain on the neck muscles. This permits the clavicular and sternal head of the sternocleidomastoïd muscle to be palpated and the top of supraclavicularis minor fossa to be marked. Moving laterally his index finger along the upper board of clavicle, the physician feels the internal clavicular insertion of the

64

trapezius muscle and marks it. A line is drawn on the skin, between the
two points. The external jugular vein can be brought into view by asking
the patient to close his lips and puff his cheeks. An "X" is marked at the
intersection of the vein with the previously traced line (figure 2).

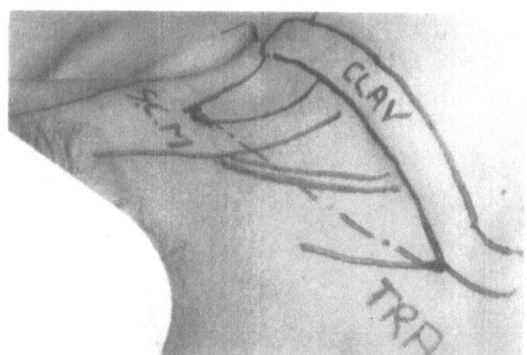

Figure 2.   Surface landmarks. From top of supraclavicular fossa
            (triangle formed by clavicle - CLAV - and the two heads
            of sternocleidomastoïd muscle - SCM)   a line is drawn down
            to edge of external clavicular insertion of trapezius
            muscle (TRA). Where this line intersects with external
            jugular vein "X" is drawn.

Procedure : the area should be aseptically prepared. An
intradermal wheal is raised at the previously determined "X" point, by
the anesthesist standing at the head of the table. A 23 gauge, 2,5 cm
needle attached to a filled 20 ml syringe is introduced through the skin
wheal and advanced slowly caudad, slighty lateral and forward, avoiding
puncture of the external jugular vein. All along the insertion, the
piston of the syringe should rest upon the auricle of the ear (fig. 3),
giving evidence of the good direction. The patient is instructed to say
"now" and not move as soon as he feels a "tingle" or "electric-like-shock"
going down his arm. When paresthesia is elicited, local anesthetic solution consisting of a mixture of 15 to 20 ml of Lidocaïne 1 % with 15 to
20 ml of Bupivacaïne 0,5 % without adrenalin, is injected after careful
aspiration. At full depth of the needle, if no paresthesia occurs and if
no other structure such as the subclavian artery or even the first rib is
encountered, redirection and reinsertion of the needle is attempted. In
our own practice, we never used a needle longer than 2,5 cm in length,
even for very corpulent patients.

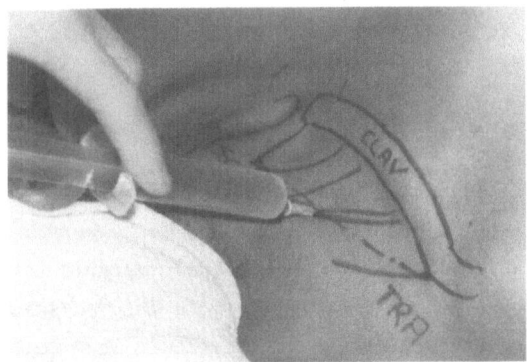

Figure 3 - Placement and direction of needle. Inserting needle, operator's hand rests upon auricle of ear. CLAV = clavicle, TRA = trapezius muscle, SCM = sternocleidomastoïd muscle.

RESULTS

In the past two years, 190 blocks of the brachial plexus, using "surface landmarks" have been performed for emergency surgery of the upper extremity. The majority of the blocks were executed during training courses by residents who were not experienced with the supraclavicular approach. Most of the patients were not premedicated, the others received a light I.V. premedication (5 mg of Diazepam). Paresthesias were elicited in all of our patients, most usually at the first attempt. General anesthesia was administered to five patients with unsuccessful blocks (2,6 %). In eleven cases, the extent of anesthesia was not complete, requiring block of the ulnear nerve and, or the median nerve. The areas not blocked were those innervated by the ulnar nerve (7 cases), the median nerve (4 cases) and the medial antebrachial and medial brachial cutaneous nerves (4 cases). The analgesia was supplemented with small doses of fentanyl (0,1 to 0,2 mg) in six cases. All the other patients (88,5 %) had complete sensory and motor block of the brachial plexus.

Complications : the left recurrent laryngeal nerve was involved in one patient who had a complete block of the brachial plexus. One patient complained of persistent paresthesias in the area of the radial nerve for three days after surgery. Horner's syndrom occured in approximately 20 % of our brachial plexus block. There were no pneumothoraces, in spite of the residents' lack of experience.

DISCUSSION

* Is the "surface landmarks" technique safe ? In a previous series (15) of 217 brachial plexus blocks performed by mostly experienced practitioners using the classical approach for supraclavicular block, the incidence of pneumothoraces was 1,5 %. With the "surface landmarks", no pneumothorax occured even though the residents were quite inexperienced. In general, the frequency of complications decreases as the anesthesiologist becomes more skilled (1, 2). Our technique avoids the practice of rib walking wich increases the risk of pneumothorax (1). Overall, the systematic use of short needles, even in obese patients may explain the absence of pneumothorax. Before us, Yasuda et al. (16) suggested inserting needles no more than 3 cm below the skin. Moore (17) recommends using a marker set, 2,5 cm from the bevel of the needle. On the other hand, the short needle length might explain that the ulnar, median, medial antibrachial and medial brachial cutaneous nerves were less frequently or more tardively blocked. These nerves originate in part from the inferior primary trunk, where, according to Lanz et al. (18), the local anesthetic arrives later and in lower concentrations.

* Are our landmarks reliable ? They are superficial and easily located just under the skin. The trapezius ans sternocleidomastoïd muscles have no important anatomic variations, which is not true of the external jugular vein. In fact, there are many variations in the origin and the termination of the vein, but the part involved in our landmarks seems to be quite consistant (19). The straight portion of the jugular vein was considered an additional guide, initially by Kulenkampff and Persky (4) and then by many other authors (1, 5, 6, 17).

CONCLUSION

Block of the brachial plexus using the "surface landmarks" seems a safe, simple to perform and successfull technique, particularly for the inexperienced physician, or when the subclavian artery is difficult to locate.

REFERENCES

1. Berry F.R., Bridenbaugh L.D.. The upper extremity : somatic blockade.
   in : "Neural blockade in clinical anaesthesia and management of pain".
   M.J. Cousins, P.O. Bridenbaugh, 1980, 296-319, Philadelphia, Lippincott Cy,
2. Moore D.C., Bridenbaugh L.D.. Pneumothorax : its incidence following
   brachial plexus block analgesia. Anesthesiology, 1954, 15 : 475-479.
3. Moore D.C., Bridenbaugh L.D., Eather K.E.. Block of the upper
   extremity. Supraclavicular approach versus axillary approach.
   Arch. Surg., 1965, 90 : 68-72.
4. Kulenkampff D., Persky M.A.. Brachial plexus anaesthesia : its
   indications, technique and dangers. Ann. Surg., 1928, 87 : 883-891.
5. Pauchet V., Sourdat P., Labat G., De Butler d'Ormont R. Anesthésie
   du plexus brachial. in : "l'anesthésie régionale", 1927, 146-168,
   Paris, Doin Ed., 4e ed.
6. Mac Intosh R.R., Mushin R.R.. Local anaesthesia : brachial plexus.
   1944, 56 p., Oxford, Blackwell Scient. Public.
7. Lamoureux L., Bourgeois-Gavardin M.. La théorie des trois perpendi-
   culaires dans l'infiltration du plexus brachial. Union Med. Can.,
   1951, 80 : 927-934.
8. Ball H.C.J.. Brachial plexus block : a modified supraclavicular
   approach. Anaesthesia, 1962, 17 : 269-273.
9. Winnie A.P., Collins V.J.. The subclavian perivascular technique of
   brachial plexus anesthesia. Anesthesiology, 1964, 25 : 353-363.
10. Vongvises P., Panijayanond T.. A parascalene technique of brachial
    plexus anesthesia. Anesth. Analg., 1979, 58 : 267-273.
11. Dupré L.J., Danel V.. Nouveaux repères pour le bloc du plexus brachial
    par voie supraclaviculaire avec une série clinique de 44 cas.
    Anesth. Analg. (Paris), 1980, 37 : 727-729.
12. Dupre L.J., Danel V., Legrand J.J., Stieglitz P.. Surface landmarks
    for supraclavicular block of the brachial plexus. Anesth. Analg.
    (Cleve), 1982, 61 : 28-31.
13. Anson B.J., Mc Vay C.B.. Surgical anatomy. 1971, tome 1, 304-313.
    Philadelphia, W.B. Saunders Ed. 5th ed.
14. Sobotta J.. Atlas d'anatomie humaine. 1977, tome 1, 168-169. Munich,
    Urban and Schwarzenberg Ed., 17th ed.
15. Dupre L.J., Guillaume F., Nandan R.M., Danel V.. Six cent treize
    anesthésies loco-régionales pendant la garde chirurgicale.
    Anesth. Analg. (Paris), 1980, 37 : 685-687.
16. Yasuda I., Hirano T., Ojima T., Onhira N., Kaneko T., Yamamuro M.
    Supraclavicular brachial plexus block using a nerve stimulator and
    an insulated needle. Br. J. Anaesth., 1980, 52 : 409-411.
17. Moore D.C.. Supraclavicular approach for block of the brachial plexus
    in : "Regional block". A handbook for use in the clinical practice of
    medicine and surgery. 1975, 221-242, Springfield, C.C. Thomas Ed.,
    4th ed.
18. Lanz E., Theiss D., Jankovic D.. The extent of blockade following
    various techniques of brachial plexus. Anesth. Analg. (Cleve), 1983,
    62 : 55-58.
19. Von Lanz T., Wachsmuth W.. Praktische Anatomie. 1955, 78-81,
    Berlin, Springer-Verlag Ed.

COMPARATIV STUDY OF THE EFFECT OF PLAIN AND CO_2-LOCAL ANAESTHETICS IN PERIPHERAL NERVE BLOCKS.

H. NOLTE [+]

In the past 15 years several publications in the international literature were concerned with the advantages of carbonated local anaesthetics over HCL-local anaesthetics. (1,2,4,5,8)

To compare these studies with the action of carbonated local anaesthetics on a single, peripheral nerve the following two studies have been carried out.

1. Blockade of the sciatic nerve at the back of the thigh
   (as described by Raj in 1972) was performed with the help of a transcutaneous nerve stimulator. 20 ml of either 1,73% lidocaine-HCL or 1,73% lidocaine-CO_2 (at a temperature of $4^\circ C$) were injected after the typical muscle twitch response. The blocks were undertaken on volunteers aged between 20 and 26.

   Analgesia was determined by pin prick, the loss of motor power with a spring loaded device and electromyography, and the difference in skin temperature between the blocked and un- blocked leg was taken as a sign of the degree of sympathetic blockade (Figure 1).

2. Blockade of the ulnar nerve was performed at the elbow with
   2 ml of either lidocaine-HCL, lidocaine-CO_2 or lidocaine with epinephrine 1 : 200.000 (at a temperature of $0^\circ C$). The blocks were performed on volunteers of 22 - 28 years of age. The experimental setup is shown and explained in figures 2 and 3. (3)

[+] Co-workers: H. Fruhstorfer, H. Petruschke, B. Roessler, U. Godt, G. Schmidt

69

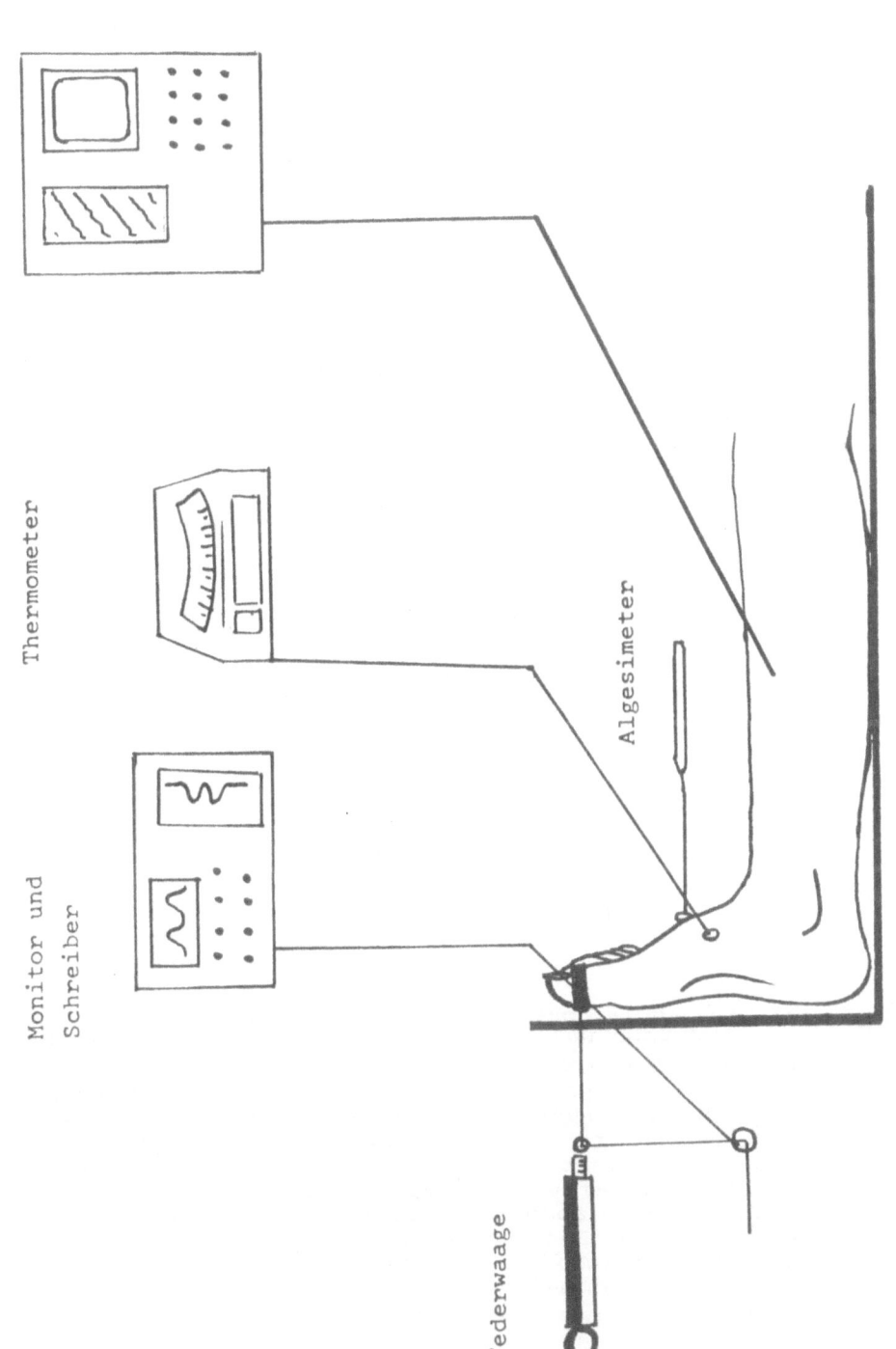

FIGURE 1

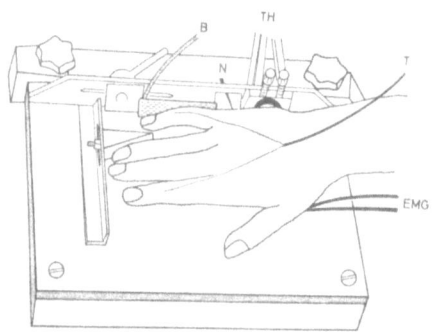

Fig. 2   Stimulating and recording apparatus. Th thermode for
cold and warm stimulation. N needle for pin prick
stimulation. B water filled balloon for measurement
of abducting force of little finger. EMG cables to
surface electrodes recording EMG of hypothenar muscle
group. T thermocouples measuring skin temperature of
little finger relative to that of index finger. Thermode, needle and balloon could be adjusted to size
and form of the hand.

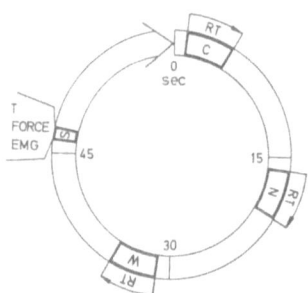

Fig. 3   Stimulus cycle consisting of four imperative stimuli
each preceded by a short warning tone pip. C cold
stimulus; N pin prick; W warm stimulus; S sound. The
subject had to press a key as soon he perceived a C,
N, or W stimulus. The reaction switched off the
stimulus and the reaction time (RT) was measured. In
case the subject did not react, the stimulus was
switched off after 4.1 sec. During the sound, the
subject had to abduct his right little finger with
maximal force. Peak force and EMG together with the
skin temperature of little finger relative to that of
index finger (T) were measured.

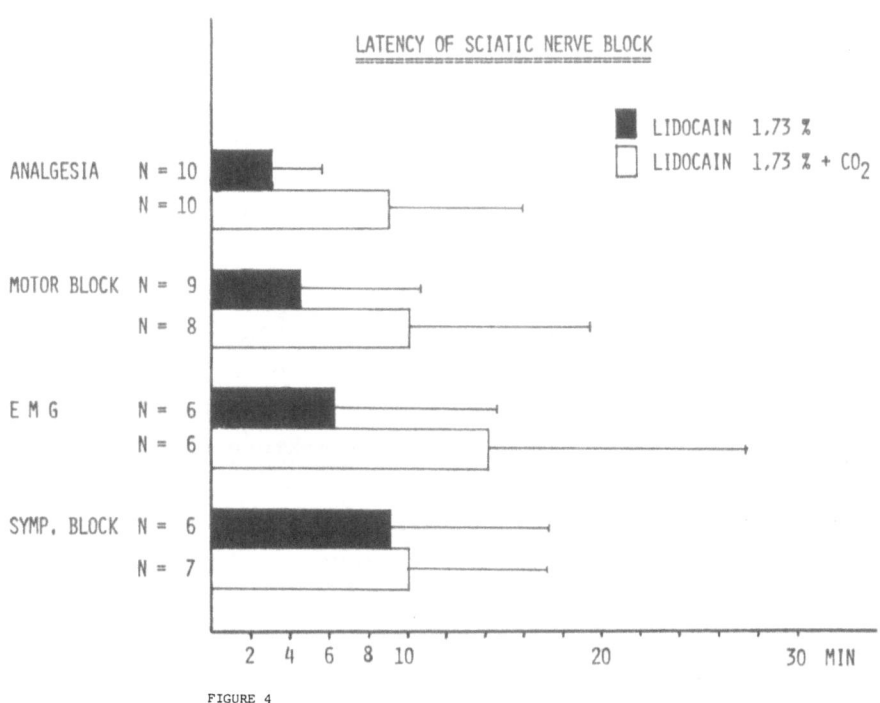

FIGURE 4

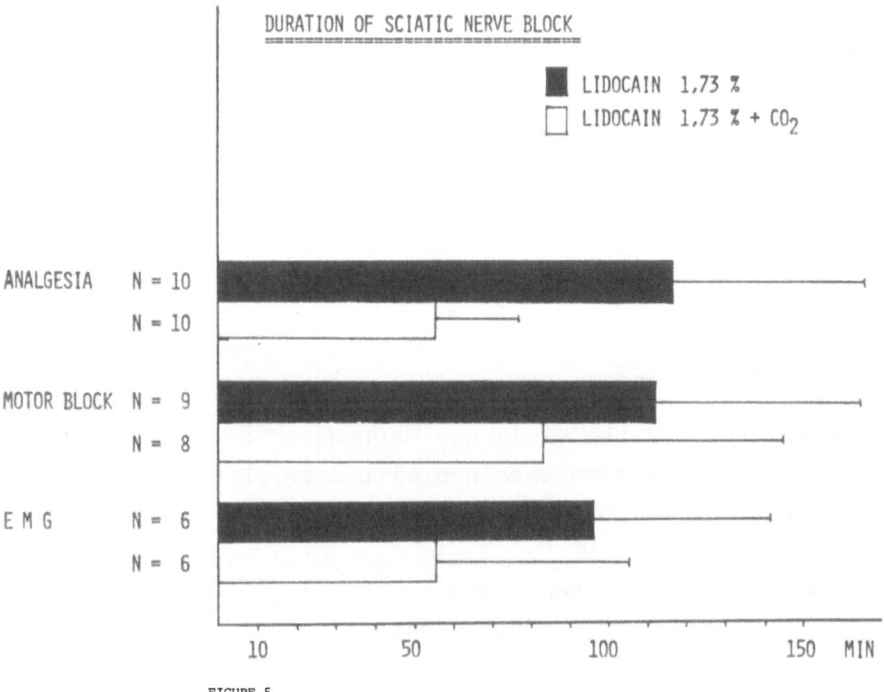

FIGURE 5

RESULTS

In figures 4, 5 and 6 the results of the blockade of the sciatic nerve are shown for the latency, the duration of sciatic nerve block, and the regression time. N represents the number of volunteers in the respective groups.

In contrast to previously published work we could not find any advantages of carbonated lidocaine in regard to latency period, duration of block and intensity of motor block. One of the reasons for these controversial results can be the fact that the solution was injected at a temperature of $4^{\circ}C$.

Following ulnar block, practically the same results as with sciatic block were found even with a more sophisticated experimental setup. With carbonated lidocaine in none of the measured parameters latency for sympatnetic block, analgesia, tactile block, warm and cold perception, and the onset of motor block, no reduction in latency could be found. The results are shown in figures 7 - 12. Only for the degree of motor blockade, carbonated lidocaine seems to have a higher success rate compared to lidocaine-HCL. As figure 12 shows, in 10 out of 12 volunteers with carbonated lidocaine, a 50% motor blockade could be found. On the other hand in only 7 of 10 volunteers who received lidocaine-HCL, a 50% motor block could be registered On the other hand, all 7 volunteers receiving lidocaine with epinephrine had a full motor block of 50% reduction in motor power.(Figure 12).

According to the duration of ulnar nerve block, there were no differences between the plain and carbonated solution. As one can expect, the solution combined with epinephrine 1 : 200.000 had a significantly longer duration of action (Figure 13).

Having obtained the same results in sciatic as well as in ulnar nerve block in a further study, the local anaesthetics were warmed up to $22^{\circ}C$, and then injected to the ulnar nerve. These results showed the opposite to the "cold" group. At room

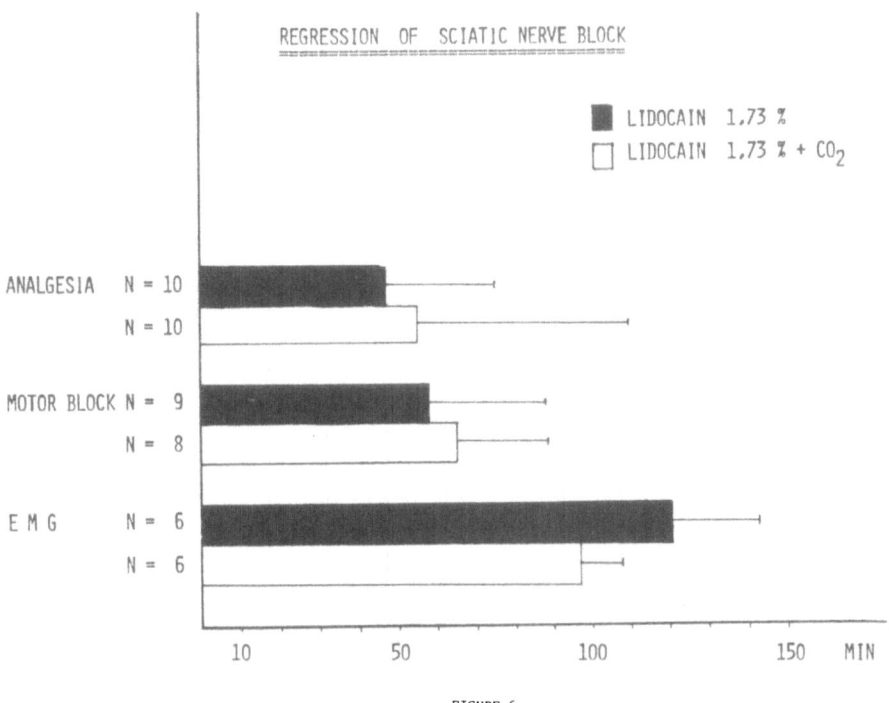

FIGURE 6

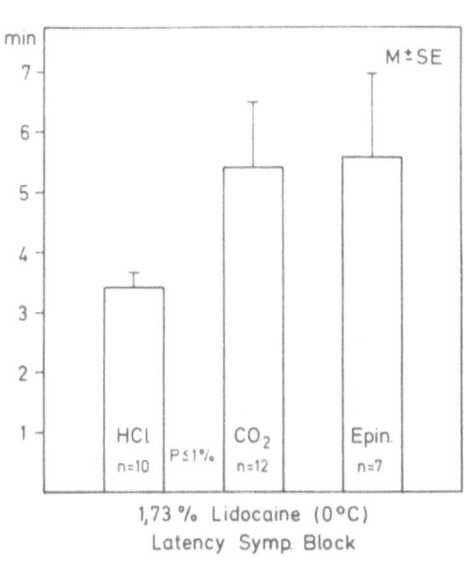

1,73 % Lidocaine (0°C)
Latency Symp. Block

FIGURE 7

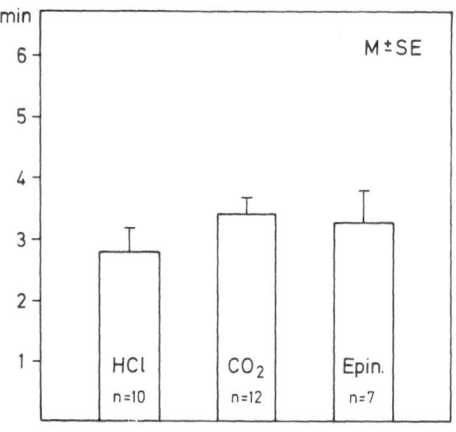

1,73 % Lidocaine (0°C)
Latency Analgesia Block

FIGURE 8

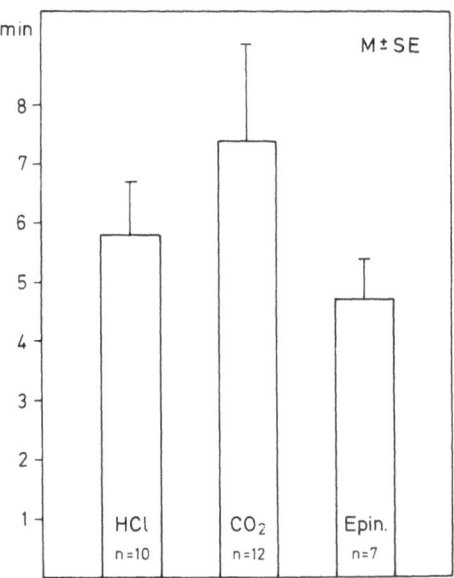

1,73 % Lidocaine (0°C)
Latency Tactile Block

FIGURE 9

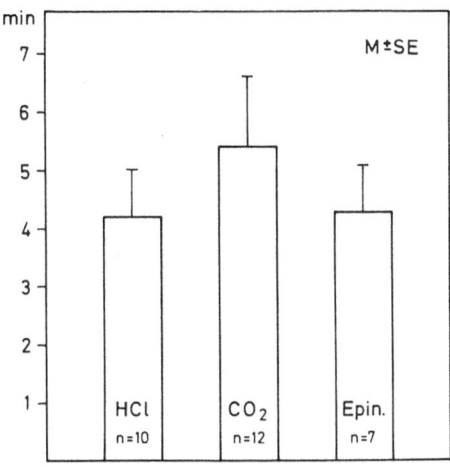

1,73 % Lidocaine (0°C)
Latency Warm Block
FIGURE 10

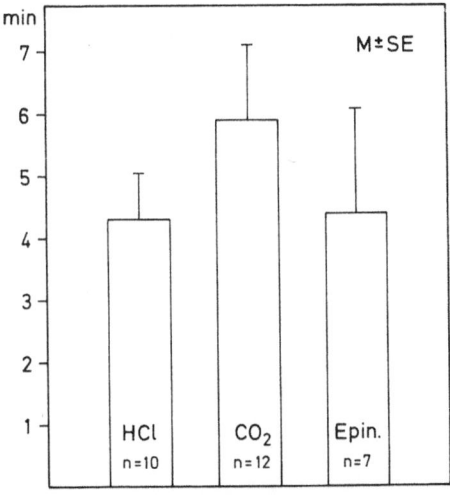

1,73 % Lidocaine (0°C)
Latency Cold Block
FIGURE 11

76

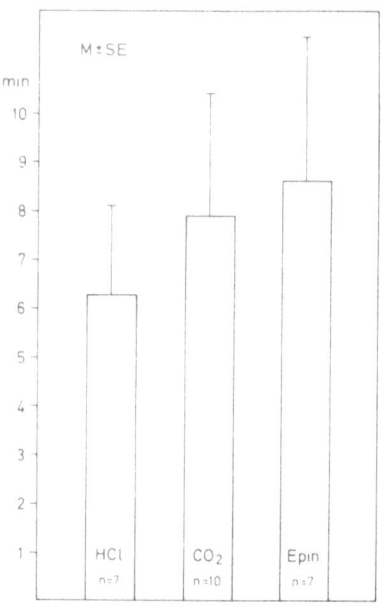

M±SE

min

1,73 % Lidocaine (0°C)
Latency 50% Motor Block

FIGURE 12

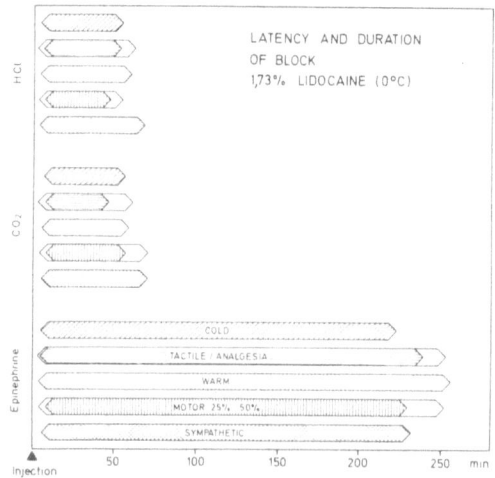

LATENCY AND DURATION
OF BLOCK
1,73% LIDOCAINE (0°C)

COLD
TACTILE / ANALGESIA
WARM
MOTOR 25% 50%
SYMPATHETIC

Injection

FIGURE 13

temperature (22°C), the carbonated lidocaine seemed to have the effect as one would expect according to previously published research. For all parameters measured the carbonated lidocaine had a quicker onset of action (Figures 14 - 19).

All results obtained did not prove statistically significant. Although the full statistical evaluation is not completed as yet, a single student-T-test showed that the statistical differences were in the 5% range.

DISCUSSION

Cold injected carbonated lidocaine did not show any differences to lidocaine HCL. Warmed up to skin temperature it seems to have the tendency of a quicker onset of action. But as in both groups no statistical differences could be shown, these results do not match up with those of the literaure. There may be many reasons for it. One may be anatomical, following the publications in recent years, all comparative studies have been performed on either epidural blocks or plexus blocks of the upper extremity. The anatomy of the epidural space, and the neural vascular sheath arround a nerve plexus is clearly different from an isolated nerve block. Thus the biochemical conditions and vascularity are different.

Another explanation for these controversal results may be the fact that by cooling the soultion the ph is increased, and thus the difference of ph of the solution to the pKa of the solution is different to those injected at room temperature. This may be responsable for changed diffusion times through the tissues for different solutions with varying temperatures and thus varying solubility of the base.

REFERENCES
1. Bromage PR, Gertel M. 1970, An evaluation of two new local anaesthetics for major conduction blockade.
   Can. Anae.J., Vol. 17, 6.
2. Bromage PR, Gertel M. 1972, Improved brachial plexus blockade with bupivacaine hydrochloride and carbonated lidocaine.

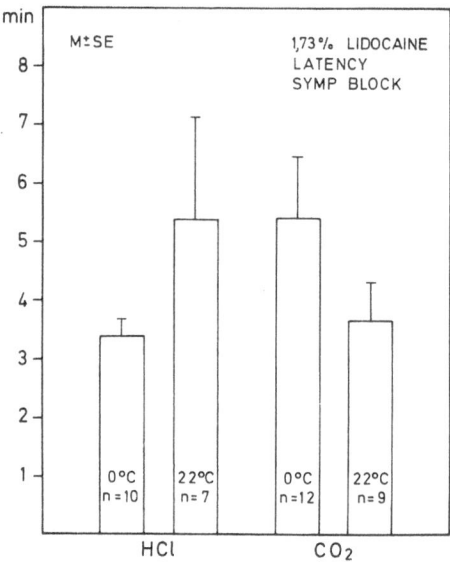

FIGURE 14

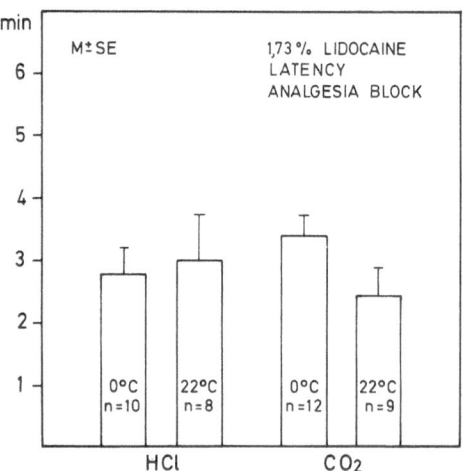

FIGURE 15

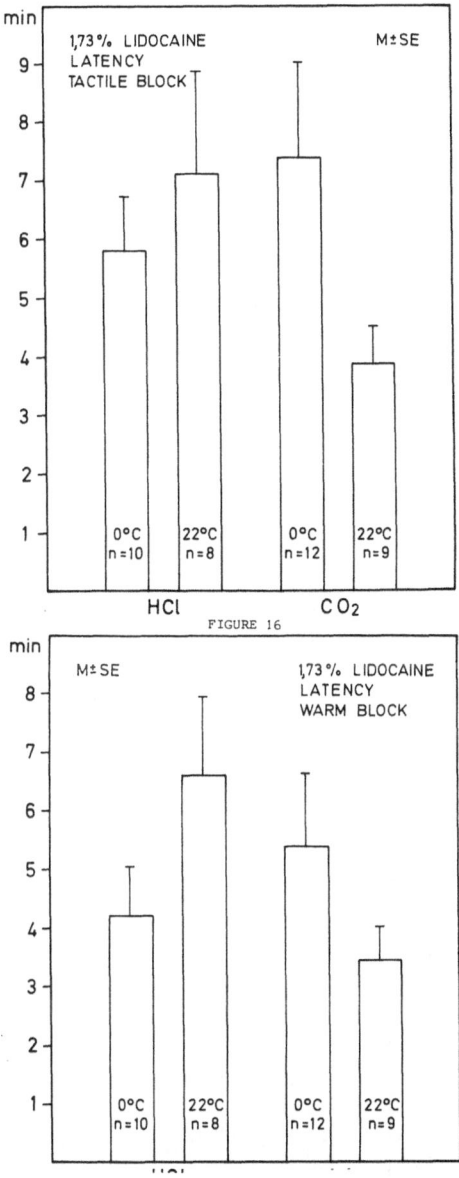

FIGURE 16

FIGURE 17

80

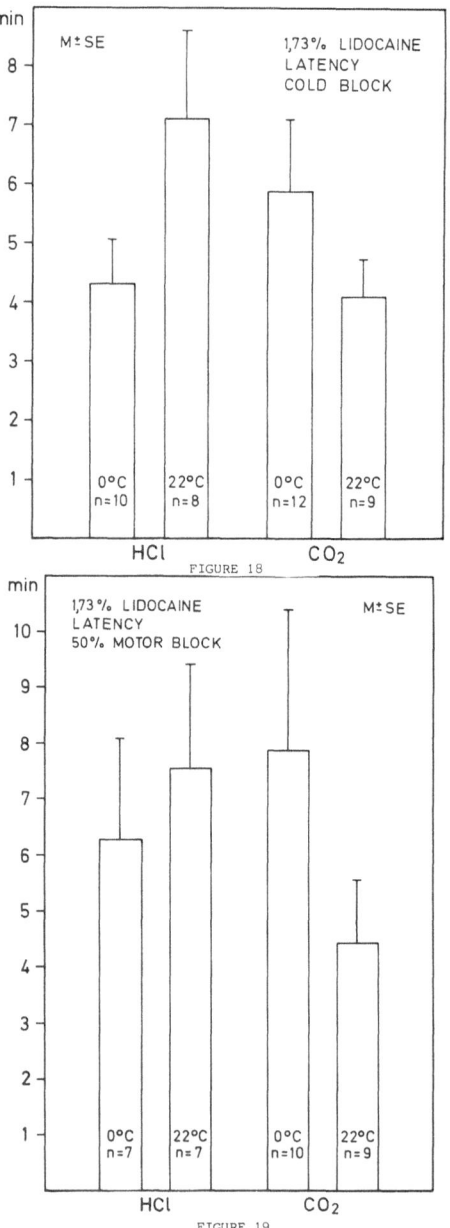

FIGURE 18

FIGURE 19

Anesthesiology, Vol. 36, 5.
3. Fruhstorfer H, Zenz M, Nolte H, Hensel H. 1974. Dissociated
   loss of cold and warm sensibility during regional anaesthesia.
   Pflügers Arch. 349, 73-82, Springer-Verlag.
4. Hartmuth J, Schulte-Steinberg O, Schütt L. 1970. Anwendung
   und Eignung der Lidocainbase-Kohlensäurelösung bei Blockade
   des Plexus brachialis. Anaesthesist, 19, 4.
5. Houle GL, Fox GS, Torkington, IMG. 1971. A comparison
   between lignocaine hydrochloride and lignocaine-carbon
   dioxide base for epidural anaesthesia during vaginal delivery. Brit.J. Anaesth. 43, 1145.
6. McClure, JH, Scott, DB. 1981. Comparison of bupivacaine
   hydrochloride and carbonated bupivacaine in brachial plexus
   block by the interscalene technique. Brit.J. Anaesth. 53, 523.
7. Schulte-Steinberg O. 1975. Heutige Indikation und Praxis der
   lokalen Betäubungsverfahren. Anaesthesiolog.Informationen,
   16, 5, 145-149.
8. Schulte-Steinberg O, Hartmuth J, Schütt L. 1970. Carbon
   dioxide salts of lignocaine in brachial plexus block.
   Anaesthesia, Vol 25, 2.

THE EXTENT OF BLOCKADE FOLLOWING VARIOUS TECHNIQUES OF BRACHIAL PLEXUS BLOCK[+]

EGON LANZ, DIETER THEISS, and DANILO JANKOVIC

1. SUMMARY

The extent of sensory and motor blockades was examined in 195 patients 5 and 20 min after four different techniques of brachial plexus block using 50 ml of 0.5% bupivacaine. The interscalene technique of Winnie (N = 50) resulted in a preferential blockade of the caudad portions of the cervical plexus and the cephalad portions of the brachial plexus. The supraclavicular approach of Kulenkampff (N = 55) and the sub-clavian perivascular approach of Winnie (N = 56) each re-sulted in a homogeneous blockade of the nerves of the brachial plexus. The Winnie modification of the axillary approach (N = 34) resulted in a preferential blockade of the caudad nerves of the brachial plexus. With all four techniques, motor blockade developed faster than sensory blockade. The difference in results suggests that the approach to be used should depend primarily upon the site of the operation. The perineural space enclosing the brachial plexus greatly faci-litates the spread of a local anesthetic when injected; how-ever, it is usually not filled completely or uniformly.

[+] This paper is based on the doctoral dissertation of D. Jankovic and on the publication in Anesth Analg 1983; 62: 55-8

2. INTRODUCTION

Winnie developed the concept of the continuous fascia-enclosed space, extending from the roots of the brachial plexus to the great nerves of the upper arm (1). He suggested that the whole brachial plexus may be blocked by one injection at any level of this space and compared this technique with epidural anesthesia. In epidural anesthesia the volume of local anesthetic will determine which nerves are blocked. The purpose of our study was to examine whether brachial plexus blocks behave similarly, that is, all parts of the plexus may be blocked with sufficient volumes independently of the approach or it is necessary to choose the approach to the plexus according to the site of operation (2).

3. METHODS

The following approaches to the brachial plexus were chosen for operations of the upper extremity:
1. the interscalene technique of Winnie (3),
2. the supraclavicular technique of Kulenkampff (4),
3. the subclavian perivascular technique of Winnie and Collins (1), and
4. the axillary technique modified by Winnie et al. (5).

The plexus was localized by eliciting one paresthesia or by electrostimulation using mono- or bipolar cannulae (6). A 50-ml sample of 0.5% bupivacaine with 5 IU ornipressine (POR-8, Sandoz Pharmaceuticals, Nürnberg, Germany) was injected at one site with an "immobile needle" (7).

Sensory and motor blockade of all upper extremity nerves was evaluated 5, 10, 15, and 20 min after injection and recorded on a chart (Fig. 1)(8). It included all sensory and motor nerves in craniocaudal order of their segmental origin. Sensory blockade was determined in the primary innervation zones by using the response to pinprick with a rating scale where 0 = sharp, 1 = dull (analgesia), and 2 = no sensation (anesthesia). Motor blockade was tested using five different nerves. The rating scale for motor blockade was: 0 = normal contraction, 1 = reduced contraction (paresis), and 2 = no contraction (paralysis).

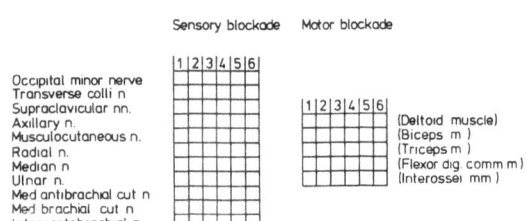

Figure 1. Chart for evaluating brachial plexus blocks. Sensory blockade is tested in the primary innervation zones of the peripheral nerves using the pinprick method. Motor blockade is determined by contraction of muscles innervated by specific nerves. The results of up to six tests are entered in the appropriate columns. See also under Methods.

Fifty interscalene, 55 supraclavicular, 56 subclavian perivascular, and 34 successful axillary approaches were evaluated. The frequencies of sensory and motor blockade of the different nerves of the upper extremity were determined for each of the four approaches. The statistical significance of differences in frequencies of the blockade of individual nerves following different approaches was determined using the chi-square test.

4. RESULTS

The four approaches examined resulted in different blockade spreads as follows:

The interscalene technique preferentially blocked the caudad nerves of the cervical plexus and the cephalad nerves of the brachial plexus (Fig. 2).

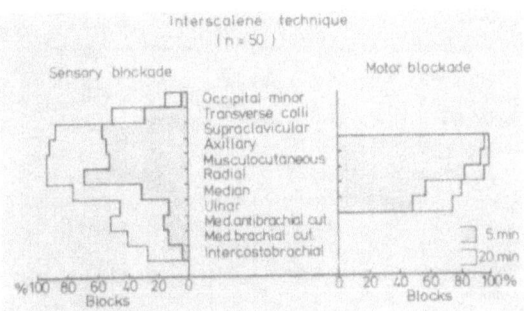

Figure 2. Interscalene technique: extent of sensory and motor blockade 5 and 20 min after injection of 50 ml of 0.5% bupivacaine.

The supraclavicular technique blocked all nerves of the brachial plexus with about the same frequency (Fig. 3).

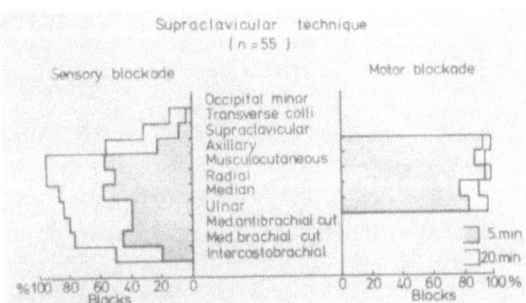

Figure 3. Supraclavicular technique: extent of sensory and motor blockade 5 and 20 min after injection of 50 ml of 0.5% bupivacaine.

The subclavian perivascular technique resulted in a similar pattern of blockade without any cephalad or caudad accents of blockade (Fig. 4).

86

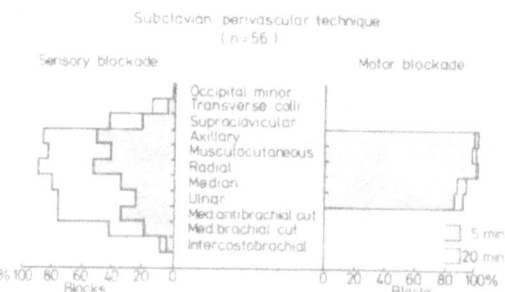

Figure 4. Subclavian perivascular technique: extent of sensory and motor blockade 5 and 20 min after injection of 50 ml of 0.5% bupivacaine.

The axillary technique preferentially blocked the caudad nerves of the brachial plexus, especially the median and ulnar nerves as well as the cutaneous nerves of the medial side of the arm (Fig. 5).

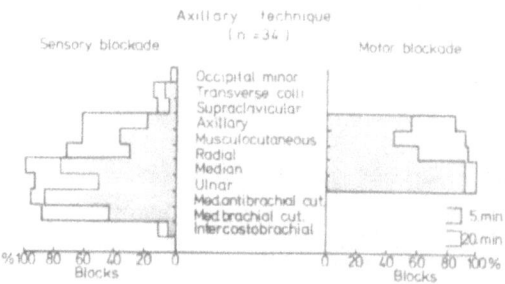

Figure 5. Axillary technique: extent of sensory and motor blockade 5 and 20 min after injection of 0.5% bupivacaine.

The interscalene and axillary techniques were associated with the widest variations in the extent of blockade (p < 0.05), whereas the supraclavicular and subclavian perivascular techniques resulted in similar extents of blockade (that were not statistically significant)(Fig. 6).

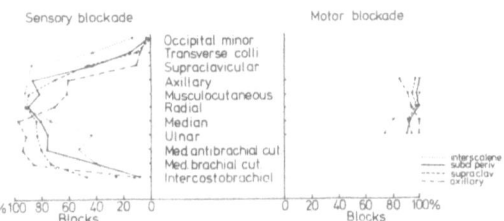

Figure 6. Profiles of the extent of sensory and motor blockade 20 min after interscalene, supraclavicular, subclavian
perivascular, and axillary techniques of brachial plexus block,
respectively. P < 0.05 between the extent of sensory blockade
following interscalene and axillary techniques; not statistically significant between the extent of sensory blockade
following supraclavicular and subclavian perivascular techniques (chi-square test).

In all instances, motor blockade developed more rapidly
than sensory blockade.

5. DISCUSSION

The differences in extent of blockade with the four approaches to the cervicobrachial plexus can be explained as
follows: the extent of blockade using the interscalene technique indicates that the local anesthetic preferentially
reaches the caudad part of the cervical plexus (C3, C4) as
well as the superior and middle trunks of the brachial plexus
(C5, C6, C7)(3, 9). The local anesthetic arrives in lower
concentrations at the inferior trunk, from which the more
infrequently blocked median and ulnar nerves originate. The
local anesthetic rarely reaches the roots of T1. The reason
for this pattern is that the local anesthetic must spread
through a large area because of the fanlike arrangement of
the trunks within the interscalene space.

The supraclavicular and the subclavian perivascular technique result in almost identical extents of blockade. In both techniques, the needle tip lies at about the same place even though it is inserted from different directions. Both techniques result in an even sensory and motor blockade of all nerves of the brachial plexus. The reasons for this pattern are that the trunks and cords are bundled closely together at the site of injection, and that the distances involved in the spread of the local anesthetic to the nerve structures are short and nearly equal.

The axillary technique results in preferential blockade of the median and ulnar nerves, less frequently, in blockade of the radial, musculocutaneous and axillary nerves (2, 10, 11). Here, the local anesthetic reaches the medial and lateral cords of the brachial plexus more readily than it reaches the posterior cord from which the radial nerve originates. The axillary and musculocutaneous nerves have a high cephalad origin.

The differences in extent of blockade resulting from use of different techniques suggest that the choice of technique should be determined by the site of operation (2), as follows:

1. The interscalene technique should be used for surgery of the clavicle, shoulder, and upper arm.
2. The supraclavicular and subclavian perivascular techniques are appropriate for surgery of the upper arm, elbow, forearm, and hand.
3. The axillary technique is best suited for surgery of the forearm and hand, especially when surgery is in the area innervated by the median, ulnar and medial cutaneous nerves.

Basing the choice of technique on the operative site (2) ensures a high probability of a successful block even when injection of the local anesthetic is made at only one site. The single injection technique has the advantage of minimizing possible neurologic damage from mechanical trauma caused by eliciting multiple paresthesias of a partially anesthetized plexus (12).

The more rapid development of motor blockade as opposed to sensory blockade was surprising, especially because we used bupivacaine. Winnie et al. (13) also observed that motor blockade developed before sensory blockade. They attributed this to the arrangement of motor fibers in the mantle and sensory fibers in the core of the trunks and cords. Thus, the local anesthetic diffuses first through the motor fibers and blocks them prior to, or simultaneously with, blockade of the sensory fibers.

The more rapid development of motor blockade makes it possible to predict the success of a block within a few minutes after injection of the local anesthetic. The evaluation of motor block is not dependent upon subjective statements made by patients, which is necessary when describing sensory block. The lack of any identifiable motor blockade 5 min after injection indicates that a successful block will probably not be forthcoming. At this point, no more time need be lost waiting for the blockade to progress.

Although we injected the considerable volume of 50 ml of bupivacaine, the extent of blockade was always dependent upon the approach used to inject the brachial plexus. The 50 ml of local anesthetic did not fill up the total perineural space entirely, and it is possible that some of the local anesthetic does leave this space. According to our findings, the perineural sheath surrounding the plexus merely gives the local anesthetic preferential direction and provides a space for spread.

The brachial plexus blocks may be compared with epidural anesthesia. The perineural space of the brachial plexus is, however, less uniformly filled by the local anesthetic than is the epidural space. In epidural anesthesia increased volumes may compensate for distal needle placement, in brachial plexus blocks they are less likely to do so. The reason may be fascial septa and leaks into neighboring fascia-enclosed spaces. Therefore the approach to the plexus

is more important with brachial plexus blocks than with epidural anesthesia.

REFERENCES

1. Winnie AP, Collins VJ. The subclavian perivascular technique of brachial plexus anesthesia. Anesthesiology 1964;
   25: 353-63.
2. Raj PP. Ancillary measures to assure success. Regional
   Anesthesia 1980; 5(1): 9-12.
3. Winnie AP. Interscalene brachial plexus block. Anesth
   Analg 1970; 49: 455-66.
4. Kulenkampff D. Die Anästhesierung des Plexus brachialis.
   Dtsch Med Wochenschr 1912; 38: 1878-80.
5. Winnie AP, Radonjic R, Akkineni SR, Durrani Z. Factors
   influencing distribution of local anesthetic injected
   into the brachial plexus sheath. Anesth Analg 1979; 58:
   225-34.
6. Theiss D, Robbel G, Theiss M, Gerbershagen HU. Experimentelle Bestimmung einer optimalen Elektrodenanordnung zur
   elektrischen Nervenlokalisation. Anaesthesist 1977; 26:
   411-7.
7. Winnie AP. An "immobile needle" for nerve blocks. Anesthesiology 1969; 31: 577-8.
8. Lanz E, Theiss D. Beurteilung der Plexus brachialis-
   Blockade. Vergleich des supraklavikularen und interskale-
   nären Zugangs. Regional-Anaesthesie 1979; 2: 57-62.
9. Vester-Andersen T, Christiansen C, Hansen A, Sorensen M,
   Meisler C. Interscalene brachial plexus block: area of
   analgesia, complications and blood concentrations of
   local anesthetics. Acta Anaesthesiol Scand 1981; 25:
   81-4.
10. Vester-Andersen T, Christiansen C, Sorensen M, Eriksen C.
    Perivascular axillary block I: Blockade following 40 ml
    1% mepivacaine with adrenaline. Acta Anaesthesiol Scand
    1982; 26: 519-23.
11. Vester-Andersen T, Christiansen C, Sorensen M, Kaalund-
    Jorgenson HO, Saugbjerg P, Schultz-Moller K: Perivascu-
    lar axillary block II: Influence of injected volume of
    local anaesthetic on neural blockade. Acta Anaesthesiol
    Scand 1983; 27: 95-8.
12. Selander D, Edshage S, Wolff T. Paraesthesiae or no par-
    aesthesiae? Nerve lesions after axillary block. Acta
    Anaesthesiol Scand 1979; 23: 27-33.
13. Winnie AP, Tay C, Patel KP, Ramamurthy S, Durrani Z.
    Pharmacokinetics of local anesthetics during plexus
    blocks. Anesth Analg 1977; 56: 852-61.

HAEMODYNAMICS AND PREGNANCY-INDUCED HYPERTENSION

M.J.N.C. KEIRSE and H.H.H. KANHAI

No complication of human pregnancy is both so common and potentially so dangerous for mother and child as the syndrome
of pregnancy-induced hypertension. Despite this, pregnant
women are almost totally ignorant of its existence. As they
feel remarkably well — symptoms generally occur very late if
not too late in the disease process — the overall significance of pregnancy-induced hypertension is not infrequently
an elusive concept to grasp. Unfortunately, that lack of understanding may even infect medical attendants who can go to
extraordinary length to explain away the hypertension and its
implications.

Although invariably reversed by delivery, pregnancy-induced hypertension is potentially far more serious than most
hypertensive states met in ordinary life. This is due to a
combination of factors of which at least three deserve particular mention. First, pregnancy-induced hypertension may
lead to some of the highest blood pressures than can be observed under any circumstances — certainly up to levels at
which arterial and arteriolar damage are expected to occur.
Second, previously normotensive or only marginally hypertensive women may achieve those excessive pressure readings over
a period of time that can be very variable but also extremely short in duration. Thus, it is hardly surprising that
some consider the condition to be very similar to that of
malignant hypertension (26). Third, although essentially a
hypertensive state, the condition can present many variable
and occasionally unexpected manifestations. These may even
dominate the clinical picture to such an extent that the re-

sulting errors in diagnosis or treatment aggravate the condition beyond repair. Unfortunately, none of the features of
the disease, not even its danger signs, are specific and that
means that alternative explanations for their occurrence are
always possible. Yet, failure to detect and appropriately
manage pregnancy-induced hypertension can still — as used
to be the case some decades ago — be lethal for either mother or child, or both.

HAEMODYNAMICS IN NORMAL PREGNANCY

Many important changes take place in the cardiovascular system during pregnancy and these have been extensively reviewed
recently by de Swiet (9). Normal pregnancy causes the systolic blood pressure to fall slightly and the diastolic pressure significantly (with about 10-15 mm Hg) within the first
few weeks; these levels remain lower until late pregnancy
when they rise again to pre-pregnancy values. Not infrequently,
this has complicated the diagnosis of pregnancy-induced hypertension. The mid-pregnancy drop in blood pressure can occur
in women with preexistent hypertension and this may lead to a
wrong diagnosis of pregnancy-induced hypertension when levels
start to rise again in the last trimester. It is not always
possible to differentiate whether the increase in late pregnancy constitutes a rise above or a return to normal pre-
pregnancy levels.

Cardiac output rises considerably during pregnancy and
views on cardiac output are a typical example of how the understanding of haemodynamic adaptations slowly evolved with changes
in technique. The classical teaching based on independent work
from, Hamilton (15), Adams (1) and Burwell (5) held that cardiac output rose slowly to a peak at 28-32 weeks after which
it declined towards non-pregnant values at term. On the basis
of these findings — and it is worth emphasizing it — count-
less patients with cardiac disease had their pregnancies ter-
minated in anticipation of this marked increase in cardiac
output that had in fact occurred a few weeks before the ter-

minations were undertaken. Presently, it is well known that
cardiac output rises rapidly in the first trimester to reach
a plateau (30 to 50 percent above the non-pregnant level) in
the first half of pregnancy which is then approximately maintained throughout (9). Thus cardiac output rises well before it appears to be needed in order to meet the demands of
pregnancy and its utero-placental circulation with a flow of
approximately 500 ml per min. Even then the increase in cardiac output with approximately 1.5 l is about three times
what would be required if all of that output were to be delivered to the uterus. Neither in time nor in magnitude
does the increase in cardiac output relate to the specific
demands of utero-placental circulation.

The rise in cardiac output is achieved both by an increase
in heart rate (with about 15 beats per min) and an increase
in stroke volume, but the proportioning is flexible and can
vary from time to time (9). Cardiac output varies greatly
during a wide range of circumstances and particularly during
labour. Even under epidural analgesia the contractions of
early labour can cause a transitory rise in cardiac output
of anything up to 2 l per min. At the onset of a contraction
about 250-300 ml — originating both from the uterus (16)
and from the relief of large vessel occlusion (18) when the
uterus lifts itself forward — are added to the circulation.
Central venous pressure may thus increase by about 3-5 mm Hg.
With little change in pulse rate most of the subsequent increase in cardiac output is an increase in stroke volume and
arterial pressure may follow the increase in central venous
pressure by about 10-20 mm Hg. Most of these changes are of
course less marked when women are in the lateral position or
given some pelvic inclination since these positions interfere
less with flow distribution between contractions. Such interference is not only due to caval obstruction — the common
cause of the supine hypotensive syndrome — for the aorta may
also be compressed by the term uterus (4). It is clear that
these factors will impede the utero-placental circulation,

but for obvious reasons there is hardly any experimental evidence about the mechanics of blood flow in the pregnant human uterus.

Since cardiac output rises early and markedly in early pregnancy, whereas arterial blood pressure does not, it follows that there must be a marked decrease in peripheral vascular resistance. This is indeed the case not only because new vascular beds are established but also because there is a general relaxation of peripheral vascular tone. This is greatest in the uterine vasculature which eventually develops in a huge bed of low vascular resistance — very similar to a large low resistance shunt. However, other organ systems especially the kidneys and skin participate in the general vasodilatation which is characteristic of normal pregnancy.

In normal pregnancy blood volume increases considerably. Most of the increase is due to expansion of plasma volume which increases with about 1250 ml in primigravid women and with about 1500 ml in subsequent pregnancies (17). Most of the rise occurs before 32 weeks of gestation with relatively little change therafter. The increase is related to the size of the fetus (24) and there are particularly large increases in multiple pregnancies (6). The total volume of red cells increases also but far less than plasma volume, which results in some degree of haemodilution in normotensive pregnancies (17).

Many of the described changes are interfered with in pregnancy-induced hypertension.

CHARACTERISTICS OF PREGNANCY-INDUCED HYPERTENSION

Consideration of the changes caused by or associated with pregnancy-induced hypertension of necessity depends on how the condition is defined. It is universally accepted that the disease is caused by pregnancy and reversed by delivery, but opinions vary widely on all other aspects including its aetiology, physiopathology and diagnostic criteria (8,23). Since pregnancy can intervene during the course of and exert

its influence on other forms of hypertension, the literature
on hypertensive states in pregnancy tends to be complex and
on occasions utterly confusing. In the past the disease was
recognized on the basis of hypertension, oedema and proteinuria
and variably known as toxaemia of pregnancy, preeclamptic
toxaemia, preeclampsia, gestosis etc. with various degrees of
severity (e.g. mild or severe preeclampsia).

Fluid retention is a normal characteristic of pregnancy
and oedema may be present in up to 40 % of normotensive
pregnancies (32). Moreover, pregnancy-induced hypertension
without oedema (dry preeclampsia) has long been recognized as
a particularly dangerous variant of the disorder (10). A
prospective study showed that the incidence of hypertension
did not differ between women without oedema and women with
early- or late-onset oedema (27). In preeclampsia without
oedema perinatal mortality is higher than in the equivalent
disorder with oedema (7), and of 43 cases of eclampsia de-
cribed by Wightman et al. (34) none had experienced excessive
water retention. Therefore, oedema is no longer recognized as
significant for the diagnosis of pregnancy-induced hypertension.
Moreover, it has little or no prognostic significance.

Central to the consideration of pregnancy-induced hypertension is the definition of hypertension which is an artificial
concept. The internationally agreed threshold of 140 mm Hg

Table I. Classification of hypertension in pregnancy

A. Pregnancy-induced hypertension
    1. Preeclampsia (mild-severe)
    2. Eclampsia

B. Pre-existent or chronic hypertension (any cause)

C. Chronic hypertension (any cause) with superimposed
   pregnancy-induced hypertension
    1. Superimposed preeclampsia
    2. Superimposed eclampsia

C. Late or transient hypertension

---

systolic and 90 diastolic is an artificial and arbitrary cut-off point. When applied to the continuous distribution of pressure readings in the pregnant population, it divides that population quantitatively and not quantitatively. For that reason, some consider an increase in blood pressure (e.g. 15 mm diastolic and/or 30 mm systolic) to be at least as important as the absolute levels (8). This is certainly considered to be an important criterion for distinguishing between pre-existent and pregnancy-induced hypertension.

The multitude of hypertensive states in pregnancy is now generally classified as indicated in table I. This also shows that the syndrome of pregnancy-induced hypertension may occur in both previously normotensive and previously hypertensive women. It does not differentiate, however, between pregnancy-induced hypertension of early or late onset, despite the fact that these may differ greatly with regard to their maternal and perinatal risks (22).

HAEMODYNAMICS IN PREGNANCY-INDUCED HYPERTENSION

Possibly, the overall picture of pregnancy-induced hypertension can best be characterized as a failure of the maternal organism to adapt to the changed physiological situation of pregnancy. Thus pregnancy-induced hypertension abolishes or diminishes many of the responses that can be considered as normal haemodynamic adaptations of pregnancy. This applies, for instance, to the increase in plasma volume (31), the ensuing haemodilution (29), the decrease in peripheral vascular resistance (11), the increase in effective renal plasma flow and in glomerular filtration rates (35). On the other hand, however, some of the normal physiological changes appear to be overaccentuated in pregnancy-induced hypertension. Thus water retention (14), sodium retention (20), reduced plasma albumin (14) and increased platelet consumption (12) are generally more pronounced than in normotensive pregnancy. For other parameters, such as maternal heart rate or cardiac output, there is generally little change when compared to

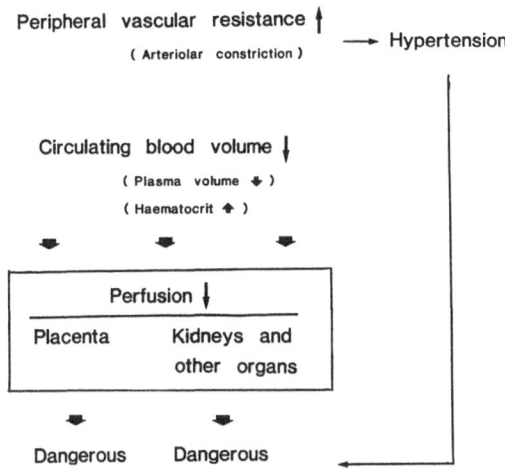

Fig. 1. Haemodynamic consequences of pregnancy-induced hypertension

normal pregnancy (2). However, when the condition is severe enough it will result in reduced cardiac output.

The direction of the changes in comparison to either normal pregnancy or its difference with the non-pregnant state is thus not systematic. This may in part explain why the pathophysiology of the condition has remained poorly understood. It also indicates that our characterisation of the condition as "a failure to adapt to the physiological situation of pregnancy" is likely to be an oversimplification.

A flow diagram of the main haemodynamic changes and their consequences are shown in fig. 1. Vasoconstriction and a greater sensitivity to pressor substances are typical characteristics of pregnancy-induced hypertension. Normal pregnant women are remarkably resistant to the pressor effects of infused angiotension II, an effect which is already noticed at the 10th week of gestation and which is also observed during pregnancy complicated by chronic hypertension. However, in women with pregnancy-induced hypertension, whether superimposed on pre-existent hypertension or not, there is a marked increase in the sensitivity to angiotension II (11). Gant and his collaborators showed that this increased sensitivity is generally present well before the increase in blood pressure occurs (11). In some cases it can be detected as early as the 22nd week of

gestation and thus many weeks (sometimes up to 18 weeks) before pregnancy-induced hypertension manifests itself.

Some consider the increased sensitivity to pressor substances as responsible not only for generalized vasospasm and
hypertension but also for the decrease in blood volume (3).
The latter would then be the consequence of a constricted
vascular compartment. Others, however, argue that the decrease
in blood volume relative to that of normal pregnancy may
preceed the onset of hypertension by several weeks (21). Which-
ever the mechanism may be, a reduced blood (mainly plasma)
volume is a characteristic feature. It is present in spite of
water retention or oedema, a fact which many clinicians presented with a bloated, oedematous patient may find difficult
to realize.

Obviously, vasospasm and reduced blood volume will exert
its effects on haemodynamics and regional perfusion of several
organ systems including kidney, liver and cerebrum. Thus, renal
haemodynamics may decrease markedly, although they will often
remain above the non-pregnant level. In severe cases, however,
oliguria and tubular necrosis may supervene. Similarly, various disturbances in liver function can occur, and these have
been described as a distinct entity among the various manifestations of pregnancy-induced hypertension (33). However, on
rare occasions they can dominate the clinical picture to such
an extent that they cloud the true pathology. The same may
occasionally apply to thrombocytopenia and disseminated intravascular coagulation, though these are more readily recognized
as a consequence of the syndrome of pregnancy-induced hypertension.

Although most of the maternal haemodynamic ill-effects
accompany the development of hypertension, effects on utero-
placental haemodynamics - or at least the basis thereof - can
preceed pregnancy-induced hypertension by several weeks if
not months. During normal pregnancy uterine blood flow increases markedly but, as mentioned above, the increase is
not temporarily related to the increase in cardiac output

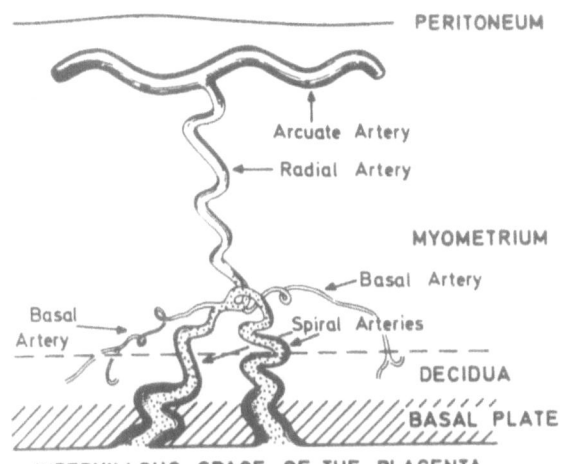

PERITONEUM

Arcuate Artery

Radial Artery

MYOMETRIUM

Basal Artery

Basal
Artery

Spiral Arteries

DECIDUA

BASAL PLATE

INTERVILLOUS SPACE OF THE PLACENTA

Fig. 2. Maternal
arterial blood
supply to the pla-
centa (28)

nor is the increase uniformly distributed within the uterus
(9). After an initial increase, flow to myometrium and decidua
do not increase to the same extent as placental flow which
reaches about 85-90 per cent of the total uterine flow at term.
The mechanism by which this is achieved may well be one of the
most ingenious haemodynamic adaptations of pregnancy, and this
is severely affected in women who are destined to develop
pregnancy-induced hypertension. As shown in fig 2, radial
arteries stem from the paired arcuate arteries that originate
from the right and left uterine arteries. These radial arteries
separate into basal arteries, which regulate flow to the myometrium, and spiral arteries, which supply the decidual endometrium and placenta (fig. 2). The spiral arteries can con-
tract and the resulting constriction close to the separating
line between myometrium and endometrium is part of the current concept of how menstruation is achieved. Early in pregnancy, however, the trophoblast invades the spiral arteries
and, by one mechanism or another, removes their musculoelastic
tissue as far back as the dividing line between myometrium
and decidual endometrium (28). That mechanism is also observed in women who later develop pregnancy-induced hypertension. However, the further wave of trophoblast migration,

which in normal pregnancy occurs at about 14-16 weeks of
gestation, appears to be absent in women destined to develop
pregnancy-induced hypertension (28). In normal pregnancy, the
trophoblast migrates along the spiral arteries up to their
origin from the radial arteries. The musculoelastic tissues
of the arteries are lost in the process and the arterial
walls are converted to wide fibrinoid tubes of low pressure
and high conductance, capable of delivering over 500 ml of
blood to the intervillous space at the end of pregnancy (19).
The latter changes apparently do not occur in women who will,
later in pregnancy, develop pregnancy-induced hypertension,
thus suggesting that haemodynamic effects in the utero-placental circulation start well before the onset of hypertension.

Table II. Causes of maternal
death in preeclampsia/eclampsia
(39 cases, England and Wales,
1973-75)

Complications	No.
Cerebral	23
Anaesthetic	5
Hepatic	4
Cardiopulmonary	3
Haemorrhage	1
Sickle-cell crisis	1
Renal	1
Hepato-renal	1

MAIN MATERNAL AND FETAL RISKS

In spite of a marked decrease in the incidence of and the
mortality ascribed to pregnancy-induced hypertension, the
British Confidential Enquiries into Maternal Deaths revealed
it to be the commonest cause of maternal death in the 1970s
(13). The cause of death is primarily cerebral (Table II) and
although several complications (e.g. oedema, thrombosis,
hypertensive encephalopathy) are described, the main com-
ponent is haemorrhage. This accounts for nearly half of all
maternal deaths from preeclampsia or eclampsia and its pa-

thology is very similar to that seen in other hypertensive states (30). This implies that hypertension is not only the defining feature of the condition, but also the principal cause of its major pathology. Nevertheless, with antihypertensive therapy the other features of the condition (abnormalities of renal, coagulation and placental function) usually persist and continue to progress in spite of lowered arterial pressure (25).

The main risks to the fetus consist of fetal growth retardation, placental abruption and fetal death in this order of severity, though not of frequency since placental abruption is the rarest of these three. Undoubtedly, all three relate to the haemodynamic changes of increased resistance in the utero-placental circulation, reduced plasma volume, and increased arterial pressure with subsequent vascular damage. However, their relative contributions are not clearly understood.

When concluding, it is worth emphasizing that, in spite of many therapeutic alternatives, no medical or other manoeuvre has so far been shown to prevent or significantly alter the ultimate course of the disease as long as the patient remains pregnant with a live fetus.

REFERENCES

1. Adams JQ. Cardiovascular physiology in normal pregnancy: studies with the dye dilution technique. Am J Obstet Gynecol 67: 741-759, 1954.
2. Assali NS, Holm LW, Parker HS. Systemic and regional alterations in toxemia. Circulation (suppl II) 30: 11-53, 1964.
3. Assali NS, Vaugh DL. Blood volume in pre-eclampsia: Fantasy and reality. Am J Obstet Gynecol 129: 355-359, 1977.
4. Bieniarz J, Maqueda E, Caldeyro-Barcia R. Compression of aorta by the uterus in late human pregnancy. I. Variations between femoral and brachial artery pressure with changes from hypertension to hypotension. Am J Obstet Gynecol 95: 795-808, 1966.
5. Burwell CS, Metcalfe J. Heart disease in pregnancy. Physiology and management. Churchill, London, 1958.
6. Campbell DM, Mac Gillivray I. Maternal physiological responses and birthweight in singleton and twin pregnancies by parity. Eur J Obstet Gynecol Reprod Biol 7: 17-24, 1977.

7. Chesley LC. Hypertensive Disorders in Pregnancy. Appleton-Century-Crofts, New York, 1978. pp 7-11.
8. Chesley LC. Hypertension in pregnancy: Definitions, familial factor, and remote prognosis. Kidney Int 18: 234-240, 1980.
9. De Swiet M. The cardiovascular system. In: Hytten FE, Chamerberlain G (eds). Clinical Physiology in Pregnancy. Blackwell Scientific Publications, Oxford, 1980. pp 3-42.
10. Eden TW. Eclampsia: A commentary on the reports presented to the British Congress of Obstetrics and Gynaecology. J Obstet Gynaecol Br Empire 29: 386-401, 1922.
11. Everett RB, Worley RJ, MacDonald PC, Chand S, Gant NF. Vascular reactivity to angiotensin II in human pregnancy. Seminars Perinatol 2: 3-13, 1978.
12. Fay RA, Hughes AO, Farron NT. Platelets in pregnancy: Hyperdestruction in pregnancy. Obstet Gynecol 61: 238-240, 1983.
13. Great Britain: Department of Health and Social Security. Report on Confidential Enquiries into Maternal Deaths in England and Wales 1973-1975. HMSO, London, 1979. pp. 21-29.
14. Good W, Hancock KW. Blood pressure, plasma osmolarity and oedema in pregnancy. Br J Obstet Gynaecol 89: 811-816, 1982.
15. Hamilton HFH. The cardiac output in normal pregnancy. As determined by the Cournand right heart catheterisation technique. J Obstet Gynaecol Br Empire 56: 548-550, 1949.
16. Hendricks CH. The hemodynamics of a uterine contraction. Am J Obstet Gynecol 76: 969-982, 1958.
17. Hytten FE, Leitch I. The Physiology of Human Pregnancy. 2nd ed. Blackwell Scientific Publications, Oxford, 1971. pp. 1-49.
18. Lees MM, Scott DB, Kerr MG. Haemodynamic changes associated with labour. J Obstet Gynaecol Br Commonw 77: 29-36, 1970.
19. McClure Browne JC, Veall N. The maternal placental blood flow in normotensive and hypertensive women. J Obstet Gynaecol Br Empire 60: 141-147, 1953.
20. Mac Gillivray I. Sodium and water balance in pregnancy hypertension - The role of diuretics. Clinics Obstet Gynaecol 4: 549-561, 1977.
21. Mac Gillivray I, Campbell DM, Jandial L. The effect of pregnancy hypertension on fetal growth. In: Van Assche FA, Robertson WB (eds). Fetal Growth Retardation. Churchill Livingstone, London, 1981. pp. 139-142.
22. Moore MP, Redman CWG. Case-control study of severe pre-eclampsia of early onset. Br Med J 287: 580-583, 1983.
23. Petrucco O. Aetiology of pre-eclampsia. In: Studd J (ed). Progress in Obstetrics and Gynaecology, vol 1. Churchill Livingstone, London, 1981. pp. 51-69.
24. Pirani BBK, Campbell DM, MacGillivray I. Plasma volume in normal first pregnancy. J Obstet Gynaecol Br Commonw 80: 884-887, 1973.

25. Redman C. Management of pre-eclampsia. In: Enkin M, Chalmers I (eds). Effectiveness and Satisfaction of Antenatal Care. Heinemann, London, 1982. pp. 182-197.
26. Redman CWG. Treatment of hypertension in pregnancy. Kidney Int 18: 267-278, 1980.
27. Robertson EG. The natural history of oedema during pregnancy. J Obstet Gynaecol Br Commonw 78: 520-529, 1971.
28. Robertson WB, Brosens I, Dixon G. Uteroplacental vascular pathology. Eur J Obstet Gynecol Reprod Biol 5: 47-65, 1975.
29. Sagen N, Koller O, Haram K. Haemoconcentration in severe pre-eclampsia. Br J Obstet Gynaecol 89: 802-805, 1982.
30. Sheehan HL, Lynch JB. Pathology of Toxaemia of Pregnancy. Churchill Livingstone, London, 1973. pp. 524-553.
31. Sibai BM, Anderson GD, Spinnato JA, Shaver DC. Plasma volume findings in patients with mild pregnancy-induced hypertension. Am J Obstet Gynecol 147: 16-19, 1983.
32. Thomson AM, Hytten FE, Billewicz WZ. The epidemiology of oedema during pregnancy. J Obstet Gynaecol Br Commonw 74: 1-10, 1967.
33. Weinstein L. Syndrome of hemolysis, elevated liver enzymes and low platelet count: A severe consequence of hypertension in pregnancy. Am J Obstet Gynecol 142: 159-167, 1982.
34. Wightman H, Hibbard BM, Rosen M. Perinatal mortality and morbidity associated with eclampsia. Br Med J 2: 235-237, 1978.
35. Wood SM. Assessment of renal functions in hypertensive pregnancies. Clinics Obstet Gynaecol 4: 747-758, 1977.

EPIDURAL ANAESTHESIA IN PREGNANCY INDUCED HYPERTENSION

Arno I. HOLLMÉN

Toxemia occurs in about 7 per cent of pregnancies mainly in
nulliparas. In severe toxemia there is a 10 per cent maternal
and 35 per cent fetal mortality. Although the cause is unknown
primary immunological disorder and uteroplacental ischemia
are the two presently accepted theories regarding the etiology.

Obstetric anaesthesia in toxemic patients has to be based
on an understanding of its pathophysiology and treatment.
High peripheral resistance and high blood viscosity increase
the cardiac work in pregnancy induced hypertension. There is
a sympathetic nervous system hyperactivity. Hypertension will
be aggravated by labour pain. Hypovolemia and hypoprotenemia
are present. Hypovolemia and especially peripheral arteriolar
constriction increase the risk of hypotension when lumbar
epidural analgesia (L.E.A.) is used and hypoprotenemia and
low colloid onkotic pressure in connection with failing left
ventricle can lead to pulmonary edema. Central nervous system
(CNS) is irritable and increase in blood pressure can lead to
convulsions. On the other hand sensitivity to all depressant
drugs in present. Imbalance in coagulation/fibrinolysis
system can lead to disseminated intravascular coagulation
(L.E.A. and bleeding!). Decreased renal and hepatic function
will modify the effects of the drugs. Placental blood flow is
decreased by vasoconstriction and intimal thickening with
fibrin deposition. The uteroplacental vessels are abnormally
sensitive to norepinephrine and angiotensin (1). The fetus is
chronically asfyxiated and will poorly tolerate any maternal
hypoxia or hypotension. Uterus is hyperirritable and sensitive

to catecholamines and placental abruption is common (Oxytocin).
The neonate is premature with severe intrauterine growth
retardation, hypoglycemia and is sensitive to drugs depressing
CNS. Drugs used to treat maternal hypertension and CNS irritability will interact with those used for anaesthesia and pain
relief (i.e. $MgSo_4 \rightarrow$ vasodilatation $\rightarrow$ L.E.A. $\rightarrow$ ris of RR $\downarrow$).

Obstetric anaesthesia should be combined with other measures
to prevent 1) hypertensive crisis (cerebrovascular accidents,
cardiac failure, abruption of placenta) 2) maternal convulsions
(maternal and fetal mortality $\uparrow$) 3) it should improve renal
and placental blood flow and 4) avoid neonatal depression. To
prevent hypertensive crises and convulsions skillful and
intensive nursing care (quiet, dark room, lateral position
and continous oxygen), proper monitoring of mother and fetus,
pharmacological means to control hypertension and nervous
system irritability are needed. To control the central nervous
system irritability magnesium sulphage or chloromethiazole
can be used. Magnesium sulphate, which is used in the USA,
also decreases uterine tone and improves the intervillous
blood flow (IBF).

To achieve efficient pain relief and prevent hypertension
lumbar epidural block producing sufficient sympathetic block
should be used. L.E.A. up to T8 level will block the passage
of impulses along the preganglionic fibers which supply
kidney, uterus and the suprarenal glands. This will decrease
the blood level of catecholamines in toxemic patients (2).
Recent observation suggests that in toxemic parturients also
the renin-angiotensin secretion can be decreased by L.E.A.
(3). Excellent pain relief, extensive sympathetic block and
humoral effects achieved by L.E.A. explains its beneficial
effect in combating continuous increase and great fluctuation
of blood and spinal fluid pressure during active labour.
Hydralazine should be used with L.E.A. whenever the diastolic
pressure increases over 100 torr. Prevention of hypertensive
crises will help to prevent convulsions as shown by Moir and
co-workers (4). To avoid post delivery hypertensive crises
L.E.A. should be continued after delivery. A parturient with

severe pre-eclampsia should post partum stay in intensive care
unit for 48 h because of continued need for antihypertensive
drugs anticonvulsants and monitoring of fluid balance.

In cases of rapidly progressing labour L.E.A. with a single
catheter technique can be used, but for labour with slow
progress the double catheter technique (with lumbar and caudal
catheters) is preferable. Before and during the commencement
of epidural block the patient's blood volume should be increased
by an infusion of lactated ringers and 25 per cent albumin
to increase CVP to 6—8 cm H_2O. This will improve the placental
blood flow, increase urinary output and decrease mean arterial
pressure (5, 6).

Maternal hypotension is the most common side effect caused
by epidural anaesthesia. Due to decreased blood volume and
general vasoconstriction toxemic patient is theoretically
prone to hypotension. It is important to avoid maternal hypotension since the fetus has a lower than normal oxygen reserve
and the intervillous blood flow (IBF) may be 40 to 60 per
cent below normal (7). Hypotension can depress the neurological
recovery of neonate during first days of life (8). Moir et
al. observed five cases of hypotension (systolic blood pressure
below 100 torr) in 150 pre-eclamptic patients treated by L.E.A.
In two of these cases the fetus died probably due to repeated
severe intrauterine hypotensive episodes. Studies about effects
of epidural anaesthesia on blood pressure (B.P.) in toxemic
patients report slight but variable decrease in B.P. (5 to 20%)
(9). Proper handling of the parturient and meticulous anaesthetic technique will minimize the risk of hypotension. It is
important to avoid aortacaval compression (lateral position)
and use carefully monitored sufficient preloading. Preferably
epidural technique includes double catheter technique.

The most flexible and least toxic local anaesthetic is
2-chloroprocaine. Use of Epinephrine with local anaesthetics
should be avoided. During slowly progressing labour 0.25 per
cent bupivacaine can be used. The injection should be given in
small repeated doses, evaluating the effect on blood pressure
before extending the block. Top-up doses should be given before

the pain reappears, which is indicated by an increase in blood
pressure. For the second stage 3 per cent chloroprocaine should
be injected through the caudal catheter. Instrumental delivery
will be beneficial because it avoids maternal pushing and the
risk for fits. However, good relaxation of pelvic floor and
excellent perineal anaesthesia are necessary for outlet forceps.
This can be achieved best by double catheter technique injecting
the local anaesthetic through the caudal catheter during the
second stage.

In severe toxemia careful invasive monitoring of circulation
(i.e., MAP, CVP) is necessary to avoid over-loading of the left
heart when fluids are administered. Hydration should only be
done in connection with vasodilatation (L.E.A.). Monitoring of
PWP would be preferable in severe pre-eclampsia (10, 11).
Studies by Joyce et al. suggest that 25 per cent albumin is the
best solution to increase CVP to 6—8 cm H_2O and avoid post
partum over-loading and pulmonary edema in pre-eclamptic
patients. In severe cases 300—400 ml was needed, whereas in
mild cases 100 ml was enough. If hypotension occurs and improved
left uterine displacement (LUD) and rapidly given infusion does
not help, ephedrine in incremental doses (2.5—5.0 mg) should be
used without hesitation.

As early as the 1940's Hingson and Edwars suggested that
L.E.A. would improve intervillous blood flow (12). The first
report of measurements of the effect of L.E.A. on placental
blood flow in toxemic patients came from Morris and co-workers
who showed an improvement of IBF (13). The first observation of
therapeutic use of epidural block to improve placental function
before labour was done in Vienna, when Janis and co-workers
(14) reported that continuous epidural block had improved the
IBF during last weeks of pregnancy in five toxemic patients.
Not only IBF but also placental function was improved by continuous epidural block. Our studies showed that epidural block
in healthy parturients will significantly improve IBF, not
depending on local anaesthetic used (15). This led to trials
looking for whether this would be true for toxemic patients,
where improvement of IBF would be of significant clinical

importance. To elucidate this problem we started a series of
studies in both primarily hypertonic and pregnancy-induced
hypertonic patients. The results showed a slight increase in
IBF after epidural block in chronically hypertonic patients,
but less so incomparison to toxemic patients. This difference
could be due to fixed type of vasoconstriction in uteroplacental
vessels in chronic hypertensive cases and normal reactivity to
catecholamines and renin of uterine vessels in chronic hypertension compared to hyperreactivity in toxemic patients (1). The
other significant finding was that segmental epidural block
using only 4 ml of local anaesthetic caused a slight (34%) mean
increase in IBF (N.S.) compared to commonly used 10 ml dose of
local anaesthetic which improved IBF significantly in severely
toxemic patients (16). These results suggest that a more extensive sympathetic bloc (T8) should be used in severe toxemia.
Decreased resistance in uteroplacental vessels due to a
decrease in blood levels of catecholamines and plasmarenin
activity as well as extensive sympathetic block may explain the
improved IBF, since we didnot observe any simultaneous decrease
in uterine perfusion pressure and muometrial tone. Recently
Campbell and co-workers studied uteroplacental blood flow using
pulsed, doppler ultrasound technique. They compared a healthy
group with a group of toxemic patients (17). In healthy
parturients the uterine arcuate arteries showed a high diastolic
flow velocity and low pulsatility indicating a low resistance
in more peripheral arteries, whereas the opposite was true for
toxemic patients. This would fit will with the hypothesis that
in toxemia there is an increased vascular resistance primarily
in the uterine spiral arteries. The technique described by
Campbell et al. would offer a new approach to study the effects
of L.E.A. on uteroplacental blood flow.

Epidural anaesthesia for Caesarean Section requires larger
amounts of local anaesthetics and significantly greater sympathetic block. This makes hypotension more common than during
L.E.A. To avoid hypotension fluid loading should be greater
than for L.E.A. Epidural anaesthesia should be used only if the
preloading with albumin (25%) will increase CVP to normal level

($\geq$ 6 cm H_2O before epidural block. A slowly acting drug (bupiva-
caine) should be used and gradual titration is important.
Maximal care should be taken to avoid aortocaval compression.
If neede ephedrine should be used.

For optimal treatment of the pre-eclamptic patient the anaesthesiologist should co-operate closely with the obstetrician.
Mortality correlates with the severity of hypertension. Anaesthetic management should aim to avoid exacerbation of maternal
hypertension. Presently epidural analgesia and anaesthesia
seems to be the best clinical practice to treat patients with
severe pre-eclampsia. The only contra-indications are maternal
coagulopathies, acute fetal distress and a mother who refuses
to have surgery while awake.

REFERENCES

1. Talledo OE, Chesley LC, Zuspan FP: American Journal of
   Obstetrics and Gynecology 2: 218-221, 1968.
2. Abboud T, Artal R, Sarkis F, Henriksen EH, Kammula RK:
   American Journal of Obstetrics and Gynecology 8: 915-918,
   1982.
3. Larva L, Hollmén A: Personal communication, 1983.
4. Moir DD, Victor-Rodrigues L, Willocks J: The Journal of
   Obstetrics and Gynaecology of the British Commonwealth May:
   465-469, 1972.
5. Joyce TH III, Loon M: Anaesthesiology 3: A313, 1981.
6. Sehgal NN, Hitt JR: American Journal of Obstetrics and
   Gynecology 2: 165-168, 1980.
7. Käär K, Luotola H, Jouppila P, Kuikka J, Toivanen J,
   Rekonen A: Acta Obstetric Scandinavica 59: 7, 1980.
8. Hollmén AI, Jouppila R, Koivisto M, Määttä L, Pihlajaniemi
   R, Puukka M, Rantakylä P: Anesthesiology 48: 350-356, 1978.
9. James FM III, Davies P: American Journal of Obstetrics and
   Gynecology 2: 195-201, 1976.
10. Benedetti TJ, Cotton DB, Read JC; Miller FC: American
    Journal of Obstetrics and Gynecology 136: 465-470, 1980.
11. Strauss RG, Keefer R, Burke T, Civetta JM: Obstetrics &
    Gynecology 55: 170-174, 1980.
12. Hingson RA, Edwards WB: Journal of American Medical Asso-
    ciation 123: 538, 1943.
13. Morris N, Osborn SP, Payling Wright H, Hart A: Lancet 2:
    481, 1956.
14. Janisch H, Leodolter S, Neumark J, Philipp K: Zeitschrift
    für Geburtshilfe und Perinatologie 182: 343-346, 1978.
15. Hollmén AI, Jouppila R, Jouppila P, Koivula A, Vierola H:
    Britisch Journal of Anaesthesia 54: 837-842, 1982.

16. Jouppila P, Jouppila R, Hollmén A, Koivula A: Obstetrics & Gynecology 2: 158-161, 1982.
17. Campbell S, Griffin DR, Pearce JM, Diaz-Recasens J, Cohen-Overbeek TE, Willson K: Lancet March: 675-677, 1983.

EPIDURAL ANESTHESIA FOR THE PREGNANT DIABETIC

Jess B Weiss

Adequate and safe anesthesia for the pregnant diabetic patient requires an understanding of the pathophysiology of diabetes in pregnancy. With this knowledge, we can apply our expertise in the provision of anesthesia in pregnancy to the diabetic, so as to minimize maternal and fetal morbidity.

Anesthestic participation and management has changed in the past decade, along with changes in the medical, pediatric, and obstetric care of these patients. The results of such changes may be seen in the vastly improved morbidity and mortality data reported from many centers.

We will examine briefly the changes in fuel metabolism during normal pregnancy and in the pregnant diabetic, the clinical course of the diabetic pregnancy, classification of diabetes, complications of diabetes in pregnancy, effects of epidural block, and modern management.

1. METABOLIC CHANGES IN DIABETIC PREGNANCY

In normal pregnancy, a constant metabolic event is the reduction of maternal glucose and amino acids because of transplacental transfer and consumption in the fetus. Both glucose and amino acids stimulate secretion of fetal insulin, while glucose also inhibits glucagon secretion from fetal islet cells.

When the amount of maternal glucose is limited, whether by starvation or diabetes, ketones made in maternal liver are readily transferred to the fetus to help meet the fetal need for fuel. Ketone bodies are also to be found in amniotic fluid.

On the other hand, free fatty acids are not transferred across the placenta to the fetus, nor does maternal insulin cross the placenta. Insulin is already present in the 12-week-old fetus, stimulated by glucose and amino acids transferred from the mother, and independent of maternal insulin supply. Thus, a fasting pregnant mother will become hypoglycemic, and go on to hypoinsulinemia and hyperketonemia. Transfer of amino acids to the fetus results in maternal hypoaminoacidemia.

Pregnancy is said to be diabetogenic, resulting from effects of placental hormones progesterone, estrogen and human placental lactogen (HPL), as well as cortisol. HPL diminishes the effect of maternal insulin, while estrogen is suggested to act as an insulin antagonist. Cortisol is increased in pregnancy, and is thought to increase glucose production in the liver and antogonize insulin action. These hormones may all cause an inhibition of pituitary growth hormone, antagonizing insulin further.

Additionally, while pregnancy causes hyperplasia of pancreatic beta cells resulting in maternal hyperinsulinemia, a diminished sensitivity to insulin has also been shown to occur. The increase in insulin appears to be a compensatory mechanism to the altered sensitivity, and so maintains glucose homeostasis.

2. CLINICAL COURSE OF DIABETES IN PREGNANCY

A variable effect of pregnancy on diabetes is seen, depending on gestational age. Early in pregnancy the primary event is transfer of glucose across the placenta to the fetus. This tends to produce maternal hypoglycemia, and may decrease insulin need. Nausea and vomiting of early pregnancy may contribute to this decreased need for insulin.

Later in pregnancy, placental hormone diabetogenic effects overcome the effects of glucose transfer to the fetus. The net result usually is an increase in insulin need by as much as two-thirds.

The tendency to ketoacidosis increases at the same time, and may reflect starvation ketosis rather than diabetic ketoacidosis, requiring glucose rather than insulin.

After delivery, the rapid fall in placental hormones and continued suppression of growth hormone result in reduction of maternal insulin needs, often to lower than prepregnancy levels.

3. CLASSIFICATION OF DIABETES

At this point, a brief look at various classifications of diabetes is in order. Their importance lies in their usefulness in predicting the outcome of pregnancy, and in individualizing patient care. Dr. Priscilla White wrote in 1978 (1), "There is hardly a subject of more importance in the study of diabetes than its prediction except its prevention or its cure."

A. The initial White classification, used worldwide, was published in 1949 (4), modified in 1965 and finally in 1977. It separates pregnant diabetics requiring no insulin (class A) from insulin-treated patients (B to F). The latter groups vary with factors present in the mother before the pregnancy, i.e. age at onset, duration of disease, and vascular complications.

B. The Pedersen classification (5) (the PBSP-prognostically bad signs in pregnancy), used since 1965, relates prognosis to factors becoming evident only during the current pregnancy (6). These indicate a poor prognosis, and include:

    1. Clinical pyelonephritis: elevated temperature and positive urine culture

    2. Precoma: diabetic acidosis with venous standard bicarbonate below 10 mmol/L.

    3. Severe acidosis: venous standard bicarbonate 10-17 mmol/L.

    4. Severe toxemia:

    5. Mild toxemia:

    6. Neglect: failure to follow recommended regimes, irrespective of cause.

The two classifications essentially make the point that prognosis depends on the diabetic and vascular state of the mother prior to pregnancy, with the added problems of the pregnancy itself.

C. Tyson and Felig (6) in 1971 designed a classification to identify the prediabetic woman, adding the immunoreactive insulin test to the usual glucose tolerance test, creating three subgroups:

    1. A-1 is glycosuria with a positive glucose tolerance and insulinopenia.

    2. A-2 is abnormal glucose tolerance with hyperinsulinism

    3. A-3 is obesity added to A-2.

D. The National Institutes of Health (NIH) classification was recommended in 1979. This recognized four major diagnostic classifications:

    1. Spontaneous diabetes--insulin dependent (juvenile onset diabetes), or insulin-independent (maturity-onset diabetes).

    2. Secondary diabetes--primary pancreatic disease, hypersecretion of insulin antagonists, drug-induced, genetic.

    3. Impaired glucose tolerance--chemical, latent, assymptomatic, or subclinical diabetes.

    4. Gestational diabetes--glucose intolerance in pregnancy - 1-3 percent of U.S. pregnancies.

4. COMPLICATIONS OF PREGNANCY IN THE DIABETIC

A variety of complications occur in diabetic pregnancy with greater incidence than in the nondiabetic. These may affect both mother and baby, involving mortality as well as morbidity.

A. Maternal mortality is no longer a major problem, except for misadventure, inadequate treatment, or ischemic heart disease as in White Class H patients.

B. Morbidity in mothers is varied in both type and incidence, and related to severity and duration of the diabetic state, as well as the extent of the chronic degenerative vascular changes. Infection, hereditary influence, obesity, and pregnancy itself are also involved. Such morbidity may be:

1. Hydramnios--commonly associated with pregnant diabetics, reported to range from 6 to 35 percent in incidence, and associated with a 13 percent rate of premature labor and delivery.(7)

2. Hypertensive disorders, notably preeclampsia, increase in incidence in diabetic pregnancy, probably due to vascular changes. Incidence has been reported from 6 to 25 percent, with most at 12 to 13 percent. Preeclampsia is one of Pedersen's PBSP's, denoting increased perinatal morbidity.

3. Edema is reported in from 10 to 22 percent of diabetic pregnancies, as a problem not restricted to the Class F diabetics with nephropathy.

4. Pyelonephritis is another of Pedersen's PBSP's, with a reported incidence up to 12 percent, higher than in nondiabetics.

5. Diabetic vascular disease, represented in White's classification as classes F, H, and R, makes such pregnancies high risk for mother or infant, although prognosis is better than it used to be. These classifications represent diabetic women with renal, myocardial, and retinal vascular disease, and are useful designations for the most serious diabetic complications of pregnancy.

a. Nephropathy is progressive in long-standing diabetics, with proteinuria, edema, and progressive renal failure.(8) Fluid retension and low renin hypertension develop. Treatment with diuretics is useful early, but as chronic renal failure sets in, dialysis and transplantation need to be considered. Hypertension is usually responsive to duretics and anti-hypertensive drugs, but may be a key factor contributing to mortality. Pedersen (9) reports a 6 percent incidence of nephropathy, while Joslin

Clinic prevalence is 9 percent. Preeclampsia may be difficult to rule out in the presence of such hypertension, proteinuria, and vasoconstriction.

      b. <u>Diabetic cardiopathy</u> manifests itself in an incidence of myocardial infarction significantly higher than in nondiabetics. There are both clinical and experimental data to support the concept of a specific diabetic cardiopathy, in addition to coronary atherosclerosis.

      There is no information available on the relationship of diabetic cardiopathy and pregnancy, and published data are scanty on coronary artery disease during pregnancy in diabetics (8). Reviews by Ginz and Husaini of acute infarction in nondiabetic pregnancies estimate an incidence of 1:10,000, with a mortality of 28 percent. Jewett in Massachusetts reviewed 784 deaths in 2,040,097 deliveries and reported 76 deaths due to heart disease. Only one of these was associated with diabetes.

      Mendelson in New York found two diabetics in 45 cases of coronary artery disease and pregnancy (10). Kitzmiller (8) in Boston reports six diabetic patients with coronary artery disease associated with pregnancy.

      c. <u>Diabetic retinopathy</u> is the most common form of vascular disease in these patients, with an incidence of 38 percent, while diabetics after 25 years of the disease have an 85-90 percent incidence. The incidence of proliferative retinopathy is estimated at 2 percent, increasing with the duration of diabetes, and found more prevalent in juvenile-onset diabetics. It is often associated with neuropathy or nephropathy.

      It has been assumed that pregnancy causes progression of retinopathy, but this has been controversial. Rodman (11) collected 201 cases of <u>background</u> <u>diabetic</u> <u>retinopathy</u> in pregnancy, found that about 10 percent progressed during pregnancy, not different than for a nonpregnant population, and concluded that such retinopathy was not ominous for the pregnant patient.

      <u>Proliferative</u> <u>retinopathy</u> is undoubtedly more dangerous. White early reported ten of 87 patients with intraocular hemorrhage, while Aiello reported six of 64 patients with progression of retinopathy and blindness in two. Laser treatment prior to or early in pregnancy seems to halt progression. An important consideration in these patients is to prevent straining, and Joslin Clinic patients with active proliferative retinopathy are advised cesarian section to prevent the Valsalva manoever in the second stage of labor.

C. Perinatal mortality

Fetal mortality is approximately twice that in the nondiabetic population, ranging from 1 to 4 percent in recent reports (7) (12), a gratifying reduction of stillbirth rates previously reported up to 12 percent. This is due at least in part to widespread emphasis on tight metabolic control, and to our increasing ability to monitor and quantitate optimal delivery time using ultrasound, L/S ratios and phosphatidyl glycerol, stress and nonstress testing of fetal heart rate, and estriol determinations.

The use of the new fetal biophysical profile is a promising technique for assessing fetal well-being. ultrasound to evaluate utilizing fetal breathing, gross body movements, tone, reactivity, and amniotic fluid volume. However, a clearer understanding of fetal pathophysiology is needed to further reduce such mortality.

Neonatal mortality has similarly decreased during this decade along with intrauterine fetal death. Pedersen (5) reported a significant decline from 22 to 7 percent perinatal mortality at Rigshospital in Copenhagen from 1946 to 1972. Major causes of mortality are respiratory distress syndrome (RDS) and congential anomalies.

However, congenital anomalies remain a major cause of perinatal mortality in diabetic pregnancies. Advances in management have had no effect on the frequency of congenital malformations in contrast to the reduction of mortality from RDS. Recent series report a range of 20 to 50 percent of all perinatal losses due to birth defects.

D. Fetal and neonatal morbidity, in addition to RDS and congenital anomalies, consists of fetal macrosomia, hypoglycemia, hypocalcemia, and hyperbilirubinemia. Excessive size for gestational age is particularly common in White class A to C diabetics as well as in prediabetics. Visceromegaly and increased deposition of fat and glycogen are found, and are attributed by Pedersen to maternal hyperglycemia, fetal hyperinsulinism and subsequent increased fetal anabolism.

A similar sequence of events has been implicated in the development of neonatal hypoglycemia, occuring in 30 to 60 percent of infants of diabetic mothers (IDM's).

Long-term morbidity beyond the perinatal period has been reported. Incidence of cerebral palsy and seizure disorders is three to five times greater in infants of diabetic mothers (IDM's) than in the general population and .may be due to maternal hypoglycemia.

Neonatal jaundice has been reported in 15 to 20 percent of IDM's. Prematurity and high hemotocrits may be causes.

Eight to 22 percent of IDM's have been reported to have neonatal hypocalcemia due to suppression of fetal parathyroids by maternal hypercalcemia.

5. EFFECTS OF EPIDURAL BLOCK IN LABOR.

An appreciation of such effects will permit knowledgeable application and skillful management of epidural so that no significant effect is seen on labor. This assumes insight into the effects on uterine contractions and the other forces of labor, utero-placental blood flow, and fetal acid-base balance.

Uterine activity and progress of labor have been extensively studied during epidural anesthesia using local anesthetics lidocaine, bupivacaine and propitocaine, with and without epinephrine (13) (14) (15) (16) (17).

Most investigators have reported a transient decrease in uterine activity involving amplitude of contractions, and lasting about 30 minutes. This occurred in oxytocin-treated women as well. Many of the studies showed significant decreases in uterine activity and duration of labor when epinephrine was added to anesthetic solutions (15) (18) (19).

The concensus is that, when the parturient is in active labor, with the presenting part engaged, with demonstrated cervical dilatation, skillful use of the technique and proper management of the patient with regard to aortocaval compression and hypotension will have no significant effect on uterine contractility or progress of labor.

Prolongation of internal rotation and the 2nd stage of labor may be prevented by using dilute local anesthetic solutions to avoid motor block of the pelvic sling, and by coaching the patient to bear down and push. Segmental analgesia is utilized during the 1st stage of labor as recommended by Bonica and others (20) to accomplish these ends.

With regard to the effects of epidural anesthesia and the increased need for instrumented delivery, there is no question that sacral segment anesthesia will interrupt the afferent limb of the perineal-diaphragmatic-abdominal reflex, and cause a loss of the urge to bear down. Again, use of a segmental block for 1st stage labor, of only analgesic local anesthetic concentrations, and coaching to bear down with contractions will minimize such need for instrumented deliveries (16).

Fetal heart rate changes with the use of epidural techniques have been the subject of many investigations. These vary greatly from being absent, to infrequent, or quite usual. Many of the reports of 10 to 40% incidence of late decelerations have been associated with the supine position, hypotension, and large doses of local anesthetic. Careful avoidance of the supine position, minimal doses of anesthetic, and prompt treatment of hypotension will reduce FHR changes changes to minimal levels (19) (21).

Adequate blood flow to the placenta is important for fetal well being, even though animal studies show large tolerances for uterine blood flow (UBF) reduction. However, the extensive sympathetic block and hypotension that can result from an extradural technique may reduce intervillous blood flow (IBF). Hollmen and his group in Finland (23) have demonstrated increased IBF using 2-chloroprocaine and bupivacaine in both normal and toxemic patients, apparently by decreasing uteroplacental vascular resistance, having earlier showed slight decreases during cesarian section. DeRosayro (23) and Albright (24) both found no significant effects on uterine blood flow (UBF) when epidural epinephrine was used in pregnant ewes and humans, with or without local anesthetic. However, Hood found significant decreases in UBF in gravid ewes given I.V. epinephrine in 5, 10, or 20 ug bolus doses, to approximate doses used in I.V. epidural test doses.

Fluid preloading, maintanence of the left lateral position, and prompt treatment of hypotension with ephedrine are necessary prerequisites for maintainence of placental flow, particularly if already compromised.

With regard to metabolic effects of epidural block in labor, many studies have demonstrated that such anesthetics decrease the degree of maternal metabolic acidosis and lactic acid accumulation usually seen, particularly during the second stage of labor when the usual "pushing" efforts are abolished by the epidural. The maternal expulsive efforts have been said to account for most of the metabolic acidosis, with probable contributions by both skeletal and uterine muscle activity, as well as by maternal hyperventilation. These metabolic changes are reflected in similar fetal changes, although maternal hypotension will also increase fetal acidemia.

From another viewpoint, UBF may well be influenced, by stress and cause fetal compromise. Maternal anxiety and pain can increase maternal catechol secretion and produce reduction in UBF. Shnider and his group (25) have demonstrated these changes in the pregnant ewe, and Abboud (26) has shown a significant drop in epinephrine levels in pre-eclamptic patients after epidural anesthesia. Buchan (27) reported reduction of the hormonal stress response to labor. Further, lower maternal cortisol levels have been found with epidural block for cesarian section compared with general anesthesia.

It has been known for over 20 years that surgical stress, general anesthesia, and trauma lead to increased endocrine and metabolic responses, such as have been demonstrated with cortisol, glucagon, catecholamines, and insulin. Afferent neurogenic stimuli are the release mechanism for such endocrine responses, and epidural anesthesia has been shown by Bromage, Cosgrove, Gordon, Kehlet, and others to inhibit such responses.

Labor and its accompanying pain certainly are to be regarded as stressful, and this has been demonstrated in both humans and animals.

6. MODERN MANAGEMENT OF DIABETIC PREGNANCY

There is no question of the reduction in perinatal mortality that has occurred in the past decade, attributable to a variety of advances in obstetric technology, and neonatology, and to better understanding of the metabolic changes of the diabetic pregnancy. The reduction has been from over 10% reported in the past 2 decades, to less than 4% in most recent series. Many reports have related reduced mortality to 3rd trimester glucose levels and tight metabolic control.

Over 25 years ago, Jorgen Pedersen showed that complications such as toxemia, hydramnios, macrosomia, intrauterine death, and neonatal hypoglycemia can be reduced by intense regulation of maternal metabolism. Since then, more aggressive metabolic regulation have been combined with advances in fetal monitoring and intensive care to reduce neonatal morbidity and mortality to present levels.

Incidence of congenital anomalies has remaind high, though information is accumulating to the effect that maternal metabolism needs to be better controlled during organogenesis, from conception through the first 7 weeks of gestation. Again, Pedersen recognized this and recommended pregnancy in diabetics only after adequate planning, involving strict metabolic control.

Miller, (28) at the Joslin Clinic, showed that elevated glycosylated hemoglobin (HBA_{1c}) levels during the first trimester related to offspring with congenital malformations. This hemoglobin measurement is related to glucose levels in the patient for the previous 4 to 8 weeks, indicating that poor control during conception and organogenesis may be involved in producing anomalies.

In addition, rat embryo cultures made hyperglycemic have resulted in neural tube defects. Such studies may hold the answer to increased incidence of malformation.

Current management is based on maintainence of plasma glucose as close to normal as possible by adjusting insulin use 2-3 time a day. Renal functior is assessed every 2 months with creatinine, BUN, and uric acid levels. Urine cultures are done each trimester, as are ophthalmologic examinations to detect proliferative retinopathy. Blood pressure is, of course, watched closely.

Fetal well-being is monitored by estriol determinations in the last trimester, on a daily basis if needed. A significant fall mandates nonstress testing, while a nonreactive nonstress test indicates an oxytocic challenge test.

Ultrasound scanning now permits following fetal movement, tone, breathing, and amniotic fluid volume, using real-time B-mode ultrasound, while fetal heart rate is recorded with a Doppler ultrasound. These techniques have allowed the creation of a new fetal biophysical profile score upon which the clinical management of the high-risk pregnancy may be based.

Use of lecithin-sphingomyelin (L/S) ratios of more than 2, and the presence of phosphatidylglycerol (PG) to indicate pulmonary maturation is helpful in determining optimal delivery time, usually 38 weeks or later.

Thus, these current practices in the medical, obstetric, anesthetic and pediatric management of the diabetic pregnancy have improved maternal, fetal, and neonatal outcome. Prognosis in these patients is being substantially improved. Perinatal mortality aproaches that of the general population, while morbidity is decreasing. The promise of decreasing the incidence of congenital anomalies has yet to be fulfilled.

REFERENCES

1. White P. 1978. Classification of obstetric diabetes. Am. J. Obstet. Gynecol. Vol. 130(2):227-230.
2. Felig P. 1977. Body fuel metabolism and diabetes mellitus in pregnancy. Medical Clinics of North American. 61:43-66.
3. Felig P., Constan D. 1982. Diabetes Mellitus. In Burrow GN Ferris TF. Medical Complications During Pregnancy. Philadelphia, W.B. Saunders.
4. White P. 1949. Pregnancy complicating diabetes. Am. J. Med. 7:609.
5. Pedersen J, Molsted-Pedersen J. 1965. Prognosis and outcome of pregnancy in diabetes. Acta endocrinol. 50:70.
6. Pedersen J. 1975. Goals and end-oints in management of diabetic pregnancy. In Camerini-Davalos RA, Cole HS, eds.: Early Diabetes in Early Life. New York, Academic Press.
7. Kitzmiller JL, Cloherty JP, Younger MD, et al. 1978. Diabetic pregnancy and perinatal morbidity. Am J. Obstet. Gynecol. 131:560.
8. Kitzmiller JL, Aiello LM, Kaldany A, et al. 1981. Diabetic vascular disease complicating pregnancy. In Clin. Obstet. and Gynecol 24:107-122.
9. Pedersen J. 1977. The Pregnant Diabetic and Her Newborn. 2nd ed. Copenhagen, Munlesgaard.
10. Mendelson CL. 1960. Cardiac Disease in Pregnancy. Philadelphia, Davis.
11. Rodman HN, Singerman LJ, et al. 1979. Diabetic retinopathy and its relationship to pregnancy. In Mirkatz JR, Adams PA (eds): The Diabetic Pregnancy. A Perinatal Perspective. New York, Grune and Stratton.
12. Constan DR, Berkowitz RL, Hobbins JC. 1980. Tight metabolic control of overt diabetes in pregnancy. Am. J. Med. 68:845.
13. Raabe N, Belfrage P. 1976. Epidural analgesia in labor. Influence on uterine activity and fetal heart rate. Acta Obstet Gynecol Scand. 55:305.
14. Schellenberg J.C. 1977. Uterine activity during lumbar epidural analgesia with bupivacaine. Am. J. Obstet Gynecol 27:26.
15. Willdeck-Lund G., Lindmark G., Nilsson B.A. 1979. Effect of segmental epidural analgesia upon the uterine activity with special reference to the use of different local anesthetic agents. Acta Anaesth Scand 23:519.
16. Jouppila R., Joupilla P., Karinem J-M and Hollmen A. 1979. Segmental epidural analgesia in labor: Related to the progress of labor, fetal malposition and instrumental delivery. Acta Obstet Gynecol Scand 58:135.
17. Phillips JC, Hochberg CJ, Petrakis JK, Van Winkle JD: 1977. Epidural analgesia and its effects on the "normal" progress of labor. Am J Obstet Gynecol 129:316.
18. Matadial L, Cibils LA. 1976. The effect of epidural anesthesia on uterine activity and blood pressure. Am J Obstet Gynecol 125:846.
19. Jouppila P, Jouppila R, Kaar K, Merila M. 1977. Fetal heart rate patterns and uterine activity after segmental epidural analgesia. Br J Obstet Gynaec 84:481.
20. Bonica JJ. 1967. Principles and Practice of Obstetric Analgesia and Anesthesia. Philadelphia. F.A. Davis, 1:616.
21. Datta S, Kitzmiller JL. 1982. Anesthetic and obstetric management of diabetic pregnant women. In: Clinics in Perinatology 9:153.
22. Hollmen AI, Jouppila R, Jouppila P, Koivula A, Vierola H. 1982. Effect of extradural analgesia using bupivacaine and 2-chloroprocaine on intervillous blood flow during normal labor. Br J Anaesth 54:837.

23. DeRosayro, AM, Nahrwold ML, and Hill AB. 1981. Cardiovascular effects of epidural epinephrine in the pregnant sheep. Reg. Anesth. 6:4.
24. Albright GA, Jouppila R, Hollmen AI, Jouppila P. et al. 1981. Epinephrine does not alter human intervillous blood flow during epidural anesthesia. Anesthesiology 54:131.
25. Shnider SM, Wright RG, Levinson G, et al. 1979. Uterine blood flow and plasma norephinephrine changes during maternal stress in the pregnant ewe. Anesthesiology 50:524.
26. Abboud TK, Sarkis F, Hung TT, Khoo SS, Varakian L, Henriksen E, Noueihed, R, Goebelsmann U. 1983. Effects of Epidural Anesthesia during Labor on Maternal Plasma Beta-Endorphin Levels. Anesthesiology 59:1.
27. Buchan PC, Milne MK, Browning MCK. 1973. The effect os continuous epidural blockade on plasma 11-hydroxy-cortico-steriod concentrations in labor. J Obstet Gynaecol Br Commonw 80:974.
28. Miller E, Hare JW, Cloherty JP, Dunn PJ, Gleason, RE, Soeldner S, Kitzmiller, JL. 1981. Elevated maternal hemoglobin A_{1c} in early pregancy and major congenital anomalies in infants of diabetic mothers. NEJM 304:22.

PERIDURAL   ANAESTHESIA   IN   CAESAREAN   SECTION

A. VAN STEENBERGE, J.L. HODY, L. FANARD

In the event of only one surgical act surviving, it should be
the Caesarean Section.
There has never been any surgery which has preoccupied so
many physicians, moralists, as well as civilian and religious
authorities and the entire world.
It saves two lives, giving a life expectancy of more than a
hundred years and is often the best guarantee of a normal
life for both mother and child.
Before the sixteenth century, Caesarean Section was only used
after women died, whereas from then on, an endeavour was made
to save the mother, the child or both of them.
Until the 16th Century, the entire birth process was left to
the midwives, more guided by religious considerations than by
obstetrical knowledge. Surgery and obstetrics, merely manual
skill, were considered vulgar and unworthy of medical science.
There was no interest in anaesthesia. Six aides were needed
to hold the patient and none to assist the surgeon.
In Africa, narcotics were given. In Europe, this was not the
case, with few exceptions, where the mother and often the
surgeon, were under the influence of alcohol before embarking
on this hazardous course. After 1847, when Simpson gave
chloroform for childbirth, this agonisingly cruel practice
ended, but the mortality rate remained.
In today's obstetrical practice, the Caesarean Section is
between four and twenty per cent of all deliveries.
Two decades ago, the average was between two and seven per
cent. The increase is partially due to a better knowledge
and understanding of the birth process. Apart from the classic
indications, foetal pathology often justifies resorting to
Caesarean Section.
Pre-term infants, delivered by the vaginal route, compared
with those born by Caesarean Section, have a significantly
higher incidence of haemorrhage. The principal cause of
morbidity and mortality in pre-term infants is cerebral
periventricular-intraventricular haemorrhage.
Computerised Tomography Scan gives an incidence of haemorrhage
of forty to fifty per cent in infants with a birth weight
below 1500 gm and an overall mortality of thirty three to
sixty six per cent.

" Aggressive" use of Caesarean Section in the delivery of all
small pre-term infants minimises perinatal asphyxia and its
consequences; planned Caesarean Section for the delivery of
the small vulnerable, very low birth weight infant is advisable.
The assumed perfect security and comfort of anaesthesia techniqu
incited many obstetricians to resort to the Caesarean Section,
sometimes from fear of medico-legal pursuits.
The present aim of the Caesarean Section is to reduce either
the risks for the mother and the foetus or substantially the
risk for one without increasing that for the other.
However, the maternal mortality rate of the Caesarean Section
is still eight times more than that in vaginal delivery,
anaesthesia being the greatest killer.
Apart from the local infiltration and spinal anaesthesia seldom
used in Western Europe, the choice remains between peridural
and general anaesthesia.
The anaesthesioligst has to select the surest method, comfortabl
for the mother, the least depressive for the foetus and giving
the surgeon the best working conditions.
Pre-term infants show greater central nervous system depression
when exposed to narcotics. It is evident that acute emergency,
without prior placed peridural catheter, requires general
anaesthesia.
The choice between general and peridural anaesthesia presupposes
that :

a. the anaesthesiologist has a thorough knowledge and experience
of peridural analgesia and anaesthesia in vaginal obstetrics and
in surgery.
b. the mother must willingly accept to remain conscious at
least until the baby is born. The presence of the father
increases confidence in the technique.
c. the obstetrician is aware of the restraints of the technique
and that he must be very gentle.

Drugs and equipment must be ready for general anaesthesia and
intubation (suction apparatus ready) at all times.

PER OPERATIVE

Peridural anaesthesia was started for Caesarean Section, now
applied in ninety two percent of all Caesarean Sections, at
the request of our obstetricians, who wanted to have sufficient
time between the induction of the anaesthesia, the incision
of the abdomen, uterus and delivery of the baby.
This mostly occured in patients with iterative sections, or
in those who had a previous laparatomy. Obese parturients
and Pfannenstiel incision also required more time.
Pfannenstiel incision is to be recommended not only for
esthetic reasons; it also contributes to post-operative comfort
and less pain, hence easier breathing, thereby reducing
pulmonary complications and wound dehiscence.

Peridural anaesthesia for Caesarean Section avoids two major causes of maternal deaths :

a.the Mendelson "syndrome", with inhalation of the stomach contents, is the major cause of death. Anti-acid therapy is not a sure protection.

b. problems with endo-tracheal intubation -failed intubation- are the second cause of maternal death.

Peridural anaesthesia reduces toxicity for mother and foetus by using a low dose of a safe agent. Bupivacaine 0.5% with Epinephrine 1/200.000, 15 to 20ml given in two sequences. The valid test dose of 5 ml slowly injected with the patient in a 5° Fowler position will indicate : if intravascular, by acceleration of the heart beat; if in the intratechal space, by the anaesthesia and the paresis of both legs within five minutes. If no such complications arise, the remaining 10 to 15 ml of Bupivacaine will be injected over a 2 to 3 minute period the patient being in a supine position, the uterus lifted and tilted to the left.With this concentration, muscle relaxation of the abdominal wall will be sufficient, as the muscles will have been stretched during the last weeks of pregnancy. After injection of the local anaesthetic agent in the peridural space, twenty minutes must elapse before the start of surgery. For good surgical condition the th4 - 5 level must be obtained. The patient must be warned that spreading the muscles, putting in the sponge and the extraction of the baby can be uncomfortable. This discomfort disappears if Fentanyl 50-100 mcg is added to the solution. The best cortical sedation is a dialogue between the anaesthe- siologist and the parents. Emotional support, focusing attention on the baby, physical massage of shoulders, holding of hand and similar distractions may carry an apprehensive patient through surgery without major complications. Gentle surgery, avoiding excessive traction on the peritoneum and uterus, eliminates discomfort and reflex nausea. Peridural anaesthesia permits the required administration of one hundred per cent oxygen to the mother, whose consumption is increased by twenty per cent, hemodilution being a constant factor. To witness the birth of her baby while undergoing surgery is a unique experience for the mother. The father is present in more than ninetyfive per cent of all sections, his presence being the best anxiolytic for the mother, unthinkable when general anaesthesia is practised. From a series of twentysix mothers who had a previous Caesarean Section under general anaesthesia and one under peridural anaesthesia, they were unanimously in favour of the peridural technique. The problem of awareness in general anaesthesia, more frequent than generally admitted and sometimes causing long-lasting psychological disorders, is of no consequences.

If for any reason, for example, foetal malformation, amnesia
is desired, Midazolam 3 mg I.V. or Flunitrazepam 0.4 mg I.V.
are the recommended drugs.
Caesarean Section should be first on schedule. All ancillary
services are also in full action for several hours.

If peridural anaesthesia is a complete failure, then General
Anaesthesia with intubation should take over. If some segments
are missed, more local anesthetic can be used if within safe
limits; if not, Ketamine I.V. in small increments (25 - 50 mg)
can be administered. As soon as the baby is delivered,
Flumitrazepam 0.2 to 0.6 mg should then be injected by I.V.
route.

The single shot technique must be avoided.

The technique is easy and simple to manage, provided it is
properly and frequently practised. Neglect of technical details
is the only cause of incidents and accidents.

SOME PRECAUTIONS

1. Two qualified persons must help the anaesthesilogist.
2. The use of a 16 or larger I.V. cannula.
3. Oxygen should be given by mask or via naso-pharyngecal
catheter.
4. A bladder catheter for continuous assessment of urine output.
5. Electro cardiography precordial lead II : arythmia detection
                                        lead V : myocardial conditio
If needed, a central venous catheter, an arterial line and
a Swan-ganz catheter.

As for the peridural technique

1. Place the peridural cannula with the patient in left
   lateral position, bending her back herself by holding her
   flexed knees with both hands,avoiding thereby caval
   occlusion.
2. The table in 15° Trendelenburg position: this favours a
   venous return in the peridural plexuses and a decreased
   pressure on the dura mater by cerebrospinal fluid.

A nick in the vessel walls or into the dura is less likely
to occur. The sitting position should not be taken.
3. A marked Tuohy needle and a marked cannula should be used
   to leave 4 cm of the cannula in the peridural space.
   Cannulas never steal into the peridural space, but slip
   easily out of it.

HYPOTENSION

The normovolemic hypotension following peridural block is the
result of concommitant sympathetic blockade, combined with
impedance of venous return.
Peripheral pooling of blood in the lower extremities and
splanchnic area along with aortocaval compression significantly
diminish the amount of venous return to the right heart.
The consequently impairs maternal pulmonary blood flow and
cardiac output with resulting maternal and foetal hypoxia.
Hypotension must always be avoided; infants poorly tolerate
the distress of diminished supply.
Therfore the uterus must be lifted and displaced to the left.
This is best done by a mechanical device or by tilting the
table 15° to the left and placing a bag underneath the right
buttock.
As hypotension is the most common phenomenon, apart from the
lifting of the uterus, crystalloids solution one litre should
be administered rapidly or, if fluid overload has to be avoided,
500 ml of a 5% solution of albumin.
Legs must be raised 15° and Trendelenburg of 10° instituted.
If these measures fail to restore normotension within a minute
Ephedrine 10 mg I.V. must be injected when normo-or bradycardia
is present. Dihydergotamine 0.5 mg I.V. should be given when
tachicardia prevails.
Reduced blood loss during peridural anaesthesia has eliminated
transfusion in more than ninetyfive per cent of all sections.
Blood loss in Caesarean Section ranges from 500 to 1500 ml.
Blood loss during incision of the abdominal wall and uterus
is in the order of 250 ml, whereas from the placental site
represents up to 1000 ml. Blood loss in a routine Caesarean
Section represents twenty per cent of the parturient's blood
volume. 1000 ml of cross-matched blood should be given if
any further blood loss is anticipated.

As soon as the baby is born, Syntocinon 5 U.I, I.V. will be
given and 10 U.I added to a 5% dextrose 1000 ml will run at
the required pace.
Ergometrine (0.25-0.50 mg) should only be used in exceptional
circumstances, when all other methods of therapy have failed.
The uterine hypertonicity drives up to 500ml blood into the
circulation.

A pronounced and lasting (3 - 4 hour) vasoconstriction causes
central venous and arterial hypertension, threatening a
cerebro-vascular rupture.

Ergometrine often induces sinus bradycardia and nodal rhythm
and causes vomiting in 65% of cases. With I.M. injection,
complications are the same, but are delayed.

POST OPERATIVE

The peridural technique provides a quiet immediate post –
operative period, as there are no respiratory tract problems,
no depression by narcotics, no sequellae of muscle relaxing
agents. As there is freedom from pain, the patient can breathe
freely and exercise arms and legs,thereby reducing deep
venous thrombosis and lung atelectasis.
Further post-operative pain relieve is obtained by peridural
injection of Bupivacaine 12.5 mg with Epinephrine and
Lofentanil 5 mcg in a 10 ml bolus. Synergism of a homeopathic
dose of the local anesthetic agents with a minute dose of an
appropriate opiate, resulted in successful pain relief, for
all mothers;60% remained pain free.
Nausea and vomiting occurred in 40% of the patients.
Itching occurred but was considered to be due to waning of
the anaesthesia. Clinical evidence of respiratory depression
was never observed.
The former alternative of injecting more local anesthetic
to provide post Caesarean Section pain relief resulted in
unfortunate consequences of hypotension and motorblockade.
Some patients resented the paresis of the legs.

All mothers took active care of their babies within twentyfour hours.
This attitude increases the mother-child relationship and
diminishes the workload of the nurses.
The gastro-intestinal transit resumes within twentyfour
hours and food intake is normal within the same period.

The hospital stay is the same as for a vaginal delivery
(eight days).

Hodgkinson showed that general anaesthesia for Caesarean
Section in parturients with pregnancy induced hypertension
produces severe bouts of hypertension during laryngoscopy,
tracheal intubation and extubation. Greater sensitivity to
angiotension and norepinephrine could be the cause. This
leads to cerebral haemorrhage or edema and cardiac failure,
responsible for 45% of all deaths associated with pre- and
eclampsia.

None of these life threatening symptoms occurs during
peridural anaesthesia.

We should like to join in his conclusion that whenever
peridural anaesthesia can be safely applied, this technique
must be our first choice. However, it will take not only
a new generation of obstetricians, but even more important,
of anaesthesiologists to introduce peridural anaesthesia in
Caesarean Section as a standard practice.

REFERENCES

CRAWFORD J.S.   Principles and Practice of Obstetric
                Anaesthesia. 1972
JAMES FR.M.   Obstetric Anesthesia: The complicated
                patient.1982
MOIR,D.   Obstetric Anaesthesia and Analgesia.
                1976
PUNDEL J.P.   Histoire de l'Opération Césarienne. 1969
OBSTETRIC ANESTHESIA DIGEST   OADIDS 1(1) 1-30 1981

EPIDURAL ANALGESIA AND HIGH RISK VAGINAL DELIVERY

JOZIEN P. HOLM

Epidural analgesia (E.A.) was first introduced in the Obstetrical unit of the State University Hospital of Groningen
in December 1978. Until that time pain relief during labour
was reached by general drugs as pethidine, pentazocine and
diazepam. The most commonly used drug was pethidine, admitted
in a dosage of 100 mg intramuscular. During the period 1973-
1980 about 20-30% of our parturients received an analgetic
and/or a sedative. Although pethidine is known as a good
analgetic, the effect on labour pain is frequently insuffic-
ient. From our own experience we learned that pain relief is
needed more in induced labour than in spontaneous labour. In
our clinic almost 100% of the induced labours are induced for
medical reasons (e.g. pregnancy induced hypertension, intrauterine growth-retardation, diabetes mellitus, post-term
pregnancy, etc.), in other words: high risk pregnancies.

PATIENTS AND METHODS

A randomized controlled study was carried out in 371
medically indicated induced labours, by simultaneous amnio-
tomy and oxytocin infusion, into the effects of intramuscular
application of pethidine and E.A. with 0.5% bupivacaine on
labour and delivery, mother and child. The effects have been
evaluated separately for nulliparae (190) and multiparae
(181). I will show you the results of the nulliparae, a group
of parturients who ask for pain relief more often than multiparae do. A group of women in labour who neither wished nor
got pain relief (N.M.-group: No Medication-group) is also
included in the comparative study. All the patients were told
about the study, and that the decision if and when pain

relief was desired would be up to them. Patients who had a
contra-indication for E.A. (coagulopathy, infections, neurological diseases, refusal of the patient to have E.A.), or
refusal to receive pethidine and demand for E.A. were excluded
Three groups were formed: 60 women who received E.A., 62 who
got pethidine and 68 who got no pain relief (Table I).

Table I. Distribution of the investigated group.

	N
E.A.-group	60
P.-group	62
N.M.-group	68

The three groups were comparable in age and duration of
pregnancy. The indications for induction of labour are shown
in Table II.

Table II. Indication for induction of labour.

Indication	E.A. (n=60)	P. (n=62)	N.M. (n=68)
Pregnancy induced hypertension/pre-eclampsia	22	22	22
Post-term pregnancy	13	23	21
P.R.O.M.	15	10	14
Abnormal ante-partum C.T.G.	1	1	2
I.U. Growth retardation	4	6	5
Others (D.M., Rh Sens., etc.)	14	9	10

The indication 'post-term' is represented relatively little
in the E.A.-group, while the indication 'others' is on the
whole represented more often in the E.A.-group. This erratic
distribution of indications did not seem to have influenced
the results. There were no significant differences in mean
birthweights. Some twin pregnancies and breech presentations
are represented in the three groups (Table III). They also
seemed not to have influenced the results.

Table III. Breech presentations and twin pregnancies.

	E.A.	P.	N.M.
Twin	2	0	1
Breech	1	2	1

TECHNIQUE OF EPIDURAL ANALGESIA

All patients received a preloading of at least 500 ml
Ringer solution or in the case of pregnancy induced hypertension, glucose 5%. The epidural space was entered in the
second interlumbar space, with the patient in left lateral
position, in the midline by the loss of resistance method
with a saline filled syringe. The epidural catheter was left
3 cm cranial in the epidural space. A test dose of 2 ml 0.5%
bupivacaine, without adrenaline, was given through the
catheter, the patient still in left lateral position. After
5 minutes another 1.5 ml 0.5% bupivacaine was given, the
patient still in left lateral position. Another 5 minutes
later the patient was asked to turn to her right side and an
additional dose of 3.5 ml 0.5% bupivacaine was given. Topping-
up doses for uterine pain were 2x3.5 ml 0.5% bupivacaine in
different lateral positions and for reaching perineal analgesia 8 ml 0.5% bupivacaine in sitting position. Patients
were told emphatically not to lie flat on their backs,
except during the second stage of labour. If there were signs
of a supine hypotension syndrome or if hypotension was
noticed after a dose of bupivacaine, a wedge pillow was used.

RESULTS

Complications of the E.A. technique have been evaluated in
100 patients (60 nulliparae and 40 multiparae) (Table IV).
In one patient it was impossible to locate the epidural
space. She could not bend her spinal column sufficiently, so
it was impossible to reach and pass the interspinal foramen.
In three patients a second insertion of an epidural catheter
was needed. In two patients because the catheter was inserted
intravasally, also after withdrawing the catheter. The third

Table IV. Complications with the technique of E.A.

	n	N	(%)
Failure to locate E.S.	*101*	1	(0.99)
Puncture vessel by needle	*103*	0	(0)
Puncture vessel by catheter	*103*	7	(6.79)
Dural puncture	*103*	0	(0)

patient had a unilateral block, the reason why a second catheter was inserted. Seven times an epidural vein was punctured by the catheter, no puncture of a bloodvessel occurred with the Tuohy-needle and there were no dural per- forations.

The analgetic effect of the E.A. was good (Table V). With 92% of our patients it was fully satisfactory. In two patients a unilateral block persisted and three patients had a persistent unblocked segment.

Table V. Effect of the E.A.

	N=100
Complete analgesia	92
Persistent unilateral block	2
Persistent unblocked segment	3
Top-ups not given correctly	2
After 5th top-up incomplete analgesia	1

In spite of preloading and of not allowing the supine position a systolic bloodpressure of less than 100 mmHg was noted 16 times after 232 doses of bupivacaine (6.9%) in 12 patients (Table VI).

Table VI. Side-effects of E.A.

	% of patients
Hypotension (syst < 100 mmHg)	12
Complete motor blockade	4
Incomplete motor blockade	19

134

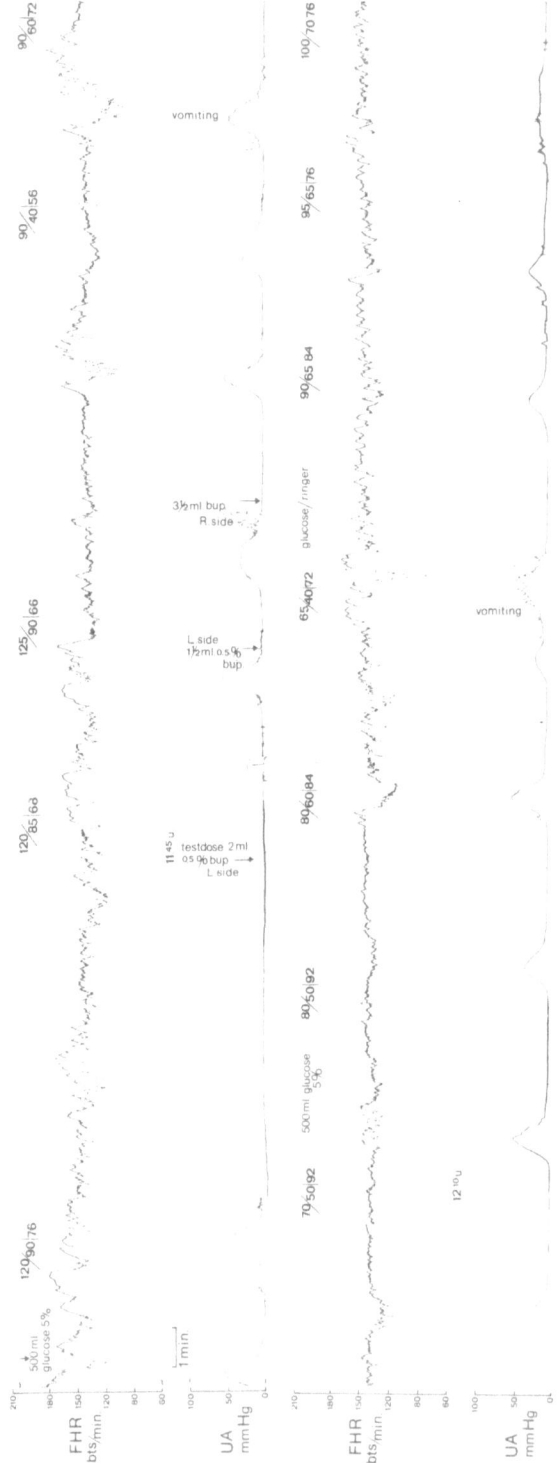

FIGURE 1. CTG of a patient with extreme hypotension after E.A.
(FHR = fetal heart rate; bts/min = beats per minute; U.A. = uterine activity in mmHg).
At the top bloodpressures and maternal pulse rate.

In all cases the hypotension was treated with extra infusion. In one patient the systolic bloodpressure dropped below 80 mmHg. The fetal heart rate pattern showed no serious signs of fetal hypoxia (Fig. 1). In one patient with hypotension the fetal heart rate pattern showed late decelerations and the fetus became acidotic. After correction of the bloodpressure the fetal heart rate pattern improved and the condition of the fetus as well (Fig. 2).

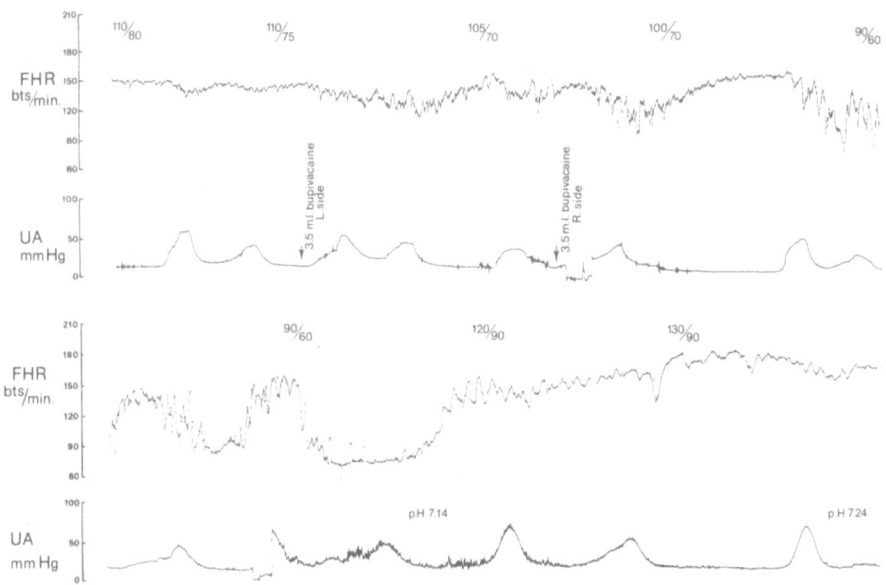

FIGURE 2. CTG of a patient with mild hypotension after a top-up (FHR = fetal heart rate; bts/min = beats per minute; U.A. = uterine activity in mmHg). At the top bloodpressures.

All the 12 children from mothers who suffered from hypotension were born with a $pH_{umb.v.}$ above 7.20. A motor blockade was noted in 23% of the patients (an incomplete blockade in 19 patients and a complete blockade in four).

The mean dosage of bupivacaine was 93.2 mg and that of pethidine 139.5 mg (Table VII). The mean dilatation at the time of the first dose was in the E.A.-group 3.1 and in the P.-group 3.5 cm. Vomiting was a frequently seen side-effect after administration of pethidine. In several patients the

Table VII. Mean dosage of bupivacaine, pethidine, top-ups,
dilatation at first dosage and top-up interval.

	E.A. N=60	P. N=62
Mean dosage bup./pethidine in mgr	93.2	139.5
S.D.	42.5	61.5
Mean number of top-ups	2.5	1.4
Mean dilatation in cm	3.1	3.5
S.D.	1.5	1.4
Range	1-7	1-7
Mean top-up interval in min	149	
S.D.	51	

the fetal heart rate pattern showed decelerations shortly
after vomiting (Fig. 3).

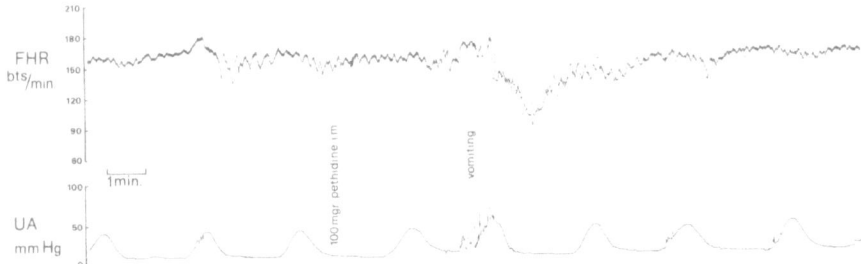

FIGURE 3. CTG of a patient who vomited after pethidine
administration (FHR = fetal heart rate; bts/min = beats per
minute; U.A. = uterine activity in mmHg).

88.3% of the patients in the E.A.-group achieved full
dilatation. In the P.-group the percentage was 88.7 and in
the group without pain relief 94.1. The duration of the first
stage of labour showed no significant difference between the
two groups under comparison (Table VIII). The first stage
was significantly shorter in the case of the group without
pain relief, which may have been the reason why no analgesia
was asked for.

There was also no difference in the mean duration of the
second stage of labour between the two groups (Table IX).
The mean duration of the second stage in the N.M.-group was
significantly shorter than in the E.A.-group. In the E.A.-
group 16 patients had a second stage beyond 60 minutes (Table X).

Table VIII. Duration of first stage of labour.

	E.A. (N=53)	P. (N=55)	N.M. (N=64)
Mean duration in hrs	8.6	8.4	6.8*
S.D.	2.8	3.7	3.4
Median	8.25	8.0	6.5
Range	2.25-16.25	3.0-17.25	2.25-21.5

*p < 0.02

Table IX. Duration of the second stage of labour.

	E.A. (N=51)	P. (N=54)	N.M. (N=62)
Mean duration in min	50.0	43.3	37.6*
S.D.	24.9	23.6	22.0
Median	50	40	31
Range	0-105	7-90	3-94

*p < 0.02 E.A./N.M.

Table X. Number of patients with a second stage > 60 min.

		E.A. (N=51)	P. (N=54)	N.M. (N=62)
sec. stage > 60 min	N	16	18	13 NS
	(%)	(31.4)	(33.4)	(21.0)

In the P.-group and in the N.M.-group the numbers were 18
and 13 respectively. It is worthwhile to note that 12 of the
51 patients in the E.A.-group received perineal analgesia
when full dilatation was reached. The mean duration of the
second stage in those patients was significantly longer than
in the E.A.-patients who did not receive perineal analgesia
at the beginning of the second stage. It seems clear that
postponing the expulsion until the fetal head is visible in
the vulva or until the bearing down reflex has fully returned,
will result in a shorter second stage period and consequently fewer instrumental deliveries, without negative effects
on the child.

Epidural analgesia nor pethidine influenced uterine
activity.

The percentages of vaginal instrumental deliveries in both groups under comparison showed no differences (Table XI). The indication for instrumental delivery in the E.A.-group seemed mostly one of time. Within this group no child in vertex position was born spontaneously after an expulsion period of more than 60 minutes, in contrast with the P.-group. The conduct with regard to that time indication has therefore influenced the frequency of instrumental deliveries.

Table XI. Vaginal instrumental deliveries.

	vaginal inst. delivery		indication time	fetal
	N	%	N	N
E.A. (N=61)	18	29.5	16	2
P. (N=62)	16	25.9	10	6
N.M. (N=69)	8*	11.6	6	2

*p < 0.05 E.A./N.M.

Considering the nature of the investigated group (women with medically indicated induced labour) it is quite plausible that the Caesarean section rate (12.1%) is high. The C.S.-percentages showed no differences (Table XII). All but one were done because there was no progress in the first or second stage of labour.

Table XII. Caesarean Section.

	N	%
E.A. (N=60)	9	15
P. (N=60)	8	12.9
N.M. (N=68)	6	8.8

Although the differences are not significant it seemed that the Apgarscores of vaginally firstborn children were worse after pethidine than after E.A. (Table XIII). The number of children with a low Apgarscore after 1 minute in the P.-group was twice that of the E.A.-group. There may be a link with the pethidine dosage.

Table XIII. Apgarscores of vaginally born children
at 1 and 3 minutes.

	E.A. (N=52)	P. (N=54)	N.M. (N=63)
Mean A.S. 1 min	8.2	7.8	8.2
S.D.	1.8	1.5	1.4
Median	9	8	8
Nr A.S. < 7	5 (9.6%)	10 (18.5%)	7 (11.1.%)
Mean A.S. 3 min	9.4	9.3	9.6
S.D.	1.4	0.9	0.7
Median	10	10	10
Nr A.S. < 7	2 (3.8%)	1 (1.9%)	0

Table XIV. Maternal pH and B.E. (mmol/l) at the beginning(1),
full dilatation (2) and post partum (3). (S.D.)

	E.A.		P.		N.M.	
	pH	B.E.	pH	B.E.	pH	B.E.
1.	7.40 *(0.05)*	-3.4 *(3.6)*	7.40 *(0.05)*	-4.3 *(2.7)*	7.40 *(0.05)*	-3.4 *(2.5)*
2.	7.40 *(0.06)*	-4.9 *(3.2)*	7.38 *(0.06)*	-6.9 *(2.6)*	7.42 *(0.09)*	-6.2 *(3.5)*
3.	7.36 *(0.06)*	-5.9 *(3.4)*	7.29 *(0.07)*	-10.2 *(3.9)*	7.31 *(0.06)*	-8.9 *(3.8)*

At the beginning of the induction, at full dilatation and
immediately after birth, a maternal and fetal bloodgas
analysis was done. At the end of the first stage the maternal
pH in the P.-group is lower, although not significantly, than
in the E.A.-group (Table XIV), while the B.E. is significantly lower: signs of metabolic acidosis. At the end of the
second stage the differences between the maternal pH, B.E.
and pO_2 in the P.-group and in the E.A.-group are significant.
In the N.M.-group the effects of hyperventilation were seen
during the first stage: a rise in pO_2 and a decrease in pCO_2
(Table XV) resulting in a rise of pH (Table XIV).

Hyperventilation is often seen during the first stage of
labour, caused by pain and by breathing instructions to
relieve pain during the contractions. Hyperventilation
results in an increase in pO_2 and decrease in pCO_2, which

causes respiratory alkalosis. Hyperventilation causes an
increase in oxygen consumption, which means less oxygen
available for other uses. The aerobic and anaerobic glyco-
lysis increases, which results in a decrease in B.E. and is
followed later on by a decrease in pH, constituting metabolic acidosis. These effects are seen during labour in the
P. and N.M.-group. It is known that hyperventilation wears
off after effective pain relief, which leads to a decrease
in oxygen consumption and lactate concentration (Sangoul '75).
Our results, i.e. less maternal metabolic acidosis in the
E.A.-group, agree with those of other investigators (Jouppila
'76, Pearson '73, Thalme '74).

Table XV. Maternal pO_2 and pCO_2 (kPa) at the beginning (1),
full dilatation (2) and post partum (3). (S.D.)

	E.A.		P.		N.M.	
	pO_2	pCO_2	pO_2	pCO_2	pO_2	pCO_2
1.	7.2	4.5	7.6	4.3	7,7	4.5
	(2.3)	(0.6)	(2.6)	(0.7)	(2.6)	(0.6)
2.	5.5	4.1	7.7	3.9	8.1	3.7
	(1.3)	(0.7)	(3.0)	(0.7)	(3.5)	(1.2)
3.	4.5	4.3	6.2	4.3	6.2	4.4
	(1.3)	(0.9)	(2.8)	(0.9)	(2.7)	(0.9)

During the second stage of labour physical exertion will
cause metabolic acidosis. The length of the second stage
will determine the degree of metabolic acidosis. It is known
that E.A. causes less maternal metabolic acidosis during the
second stage (Pearson '73, Thalme '74, Zador '74). Our
investigation confirms these findings.

The vaginally firstborn children in the E.A.-group, too,
showed less metabolic acidosis after birth than the children
in the P.-group in particular, but in the N.M.-group as well
(Table XVI). Most likely the higher incidence of metabolic
acidosis with children in the P.-group is the result of the
higher incidence of maternal metabolic acidosis.

A survey of the most important results indicates a lower
pH and B.E. in the umbilical artery and vein in the P.-group
of vaginally born children as the only significant difference.

Table XVI. Fetal pH and B.E. (mmol/l) at the beginning (1), full dilatation (2) and post partum (3) (S.D.)

	E.A. pH	E.A. B.E.	P. pH	P. B.E.	N.M. pH	N.M. B.E.
1.	7.32	-2.3	7.32	-2.8	7.32	-3.4
	(0.04)	(3.7)	(0.04)	(3.1)	(0.04)	(2.9)
2.	7.32	-2.1	7.28	-5.4	7.32	-2.7
	(0.05)	(3.5)	(0.06)	(4.2)	(0.06)	(3.7)
3. u.a.	7.24	-6.7	7.16	-10.0	7.21	-8.2
	(0.07)	(3.7)	(0.08)	(4.9)	(0.06)	(4.2)
u.v.	7.31	-5.6	7.23	-8.6	7.28	-6.9
	(0.07)	(3.2)	(0.07)	(4.3)	(0.07)	(3.4)

The investigation not only justifies the use of E.A. with cases of medically indicated induced labour when pain relief is desired, but E.A. also appears to be superior as far as analgetic effect and occurrence of metabolic acidosis in the case of firstborn children is concerned, to pethidine, the analgetic drug most frequently used during labour in the Netherlands.

REFERENCES

1. Joupilla R, Hollmén A. 1976. The effect of segmental epidural analgesia on maternal and foetal acid-base balance, lactate, serum potassium and creatine phosphokinase during labour. Acta Anaesth. Scand. 20:259.
2. Pearson JF, Davies P. 1973. The effect of continuous lumbar epidural analgesia on the acid-base status of maternal arterial blood during the first stage of labour. J. Obstet. Gynaecol. Br. Cwlth. 80:218.
3. Pearson JF, Davies P. 1973. The effect of continuous lumbar epidural analgesia on maternal acid-base balance and arterial lactate concentration during the second stage of labour. J. Obstet. Gynaecol. Br. Cwlth. 80:225.
4. Thalme B, Belfrage P, Raabe N. 1974. Lumbar epidural analgesia in labour. I: Acid-base balance and clinical condition of mother, fetus and newborn child. Acta Obstet Gynecol. Scand. 53:27.
5. Zador G. 1974. Continuous lumbar epidural analgesia and pudendal block for vaginal delivery. Effects on the mother, foetus and uterine activity using lidocaine in different dosage forms. Acta Obstet. Gynecol. Scand. 534.

CONCEPTS AND PERSPECTIVES IN SPINAL ANESTHESIA
Nicholas M. Greene

The recent renaissance of spinal anesthesia is due, in no small
part, to two factors. First is increased awareness of what the
physiologic responses to spinal anesthesia consist of, especially
cardiovascular responses. Second is the development of new concepts in
cardiovascular physiology, especially appreciation of factors involved
in regulation of myocardial oxygenation. To realize the full potential
of spinal anesthesia requires full understanding of how and why spinal
anesthesia affects cardiovascular function and what the cardiovascular
responses to spinal anesthesia mean in terms of myocardial oxygenation
(1).

The effects of spinal anesthesia on cardiovascular function are
mediated entirely by the preganglionic sympathetic denervation produced
by injection of local anesthetic solutions into the subarachnoid
space. Concentrations of drugs used in spinal anesthesia, local
anesthetics as well as vasoconstrictors, are too low in peripheral
blood to produce systemic pharmacologic responses. Study of
cardiovascular responses to spinal anesthesia becomes a study of
cardiovascular responses to pure sympathetic denervation. Spinal
anesthesia thus differs from other forms of major regional anesthesia,
including epidural anesthesia. The latter are associated with
pharmacologically active blood concentrations of local anesthetics
and/or vasoconstrictors sufficient to significantly alter the
cardiovascular responses produced by pure preganglionic sympathetic
denervation.

The magnitude of cardiovascular responses to spinal anesthesia is a
function of the degree to which symathetic outflow is blocked. The
local anesthetic in the subarachnoid space that blocks sympathetic
outflow also blocks somatic sensory fibers. There is, however, no
clear-cut relationship between the extent of sensory denervation, i.e.
height of spinal anesthesia, and the magnitude of changes in
cardiovascular function. The absence of such a clear-cut relationship
is the result of four factors. First, preganglionic sympathetic fibers

ascend and descend in the paravertebral sympathetic chain before synapsing in the paravertebral sympathetic ganglia with as many as five or even six postganglionic sympathetic fibers. Block of a single preganglionic fiber is therefore associated with a diffuse peripheral sympathetic response extending well beyond the somatic sensory dermatome level at which the preganglionic fiber is blocked. Block (or stimulation) of a preganglionic sympathetic fiber at, for example, the level of T_6 produces peripheral responses in sensory dermatomes T_{4-8}. Peripheral changes in sympathetic activity during spinal anesthesia may be unexpectedly diffuse and widespread.

Second, a zone of differential sympathetic blockade develops during spinal anesthesia. It arises for two reasons. The concentration of local anesthetic in cerebrospinal fluid decreases as a function of distance from the site of injection. And, second, smaller nerve fibers (e.g. preganglionic sympathetic fibers) are more sensitive to local anesthetics than are larger fibers (e.g. somatic sensory fibers). The level of preganglionic sympathetic denervation during spinal anesthesia averages two spinal segmental levels higher than the level of somatic sensory denervation during hyperbaric spinal anesthesia. The zone of differential sympathetic blockade may, however, be as great as six spinal segments. The level of sympathetic denervation is therefore greater than expected on the basis of the level of sensory denervation.

Third, the zone of differential sympathetic blockade means that a T_3 level of sensory anesthesia is, since the highest preganglionic sympathetic fiber arises at the level of T_1, associated with total sympathetic denervation. Since sympathetic denervation is complete with a sensory level of T_3, mid-cervical levels of sensory anesthesia are associated with no greater cardiovascular responses than are T_3 levels.

And, fourth, in the presence of preganglionic sympathetic denervation that is less than complete during spinal anesthesia, reflex increase in sympathetic activity in sympathetically intact areas partially compensates for cardiovascular changes produced by loss of sympathetic tone in sympathetically denervated areas.

Cardiovascular responses to sympathetic denervation produced by spinal anesthesia are characterized by peripheral vasodilation. On the arterial side, this includes arterial and, physiologically substantially more important, arteriolar vasodilation. The result of vasodilation on the arterial side of the circulation is the well known decrease in systemic vascular resistance, i.e. left ventricular afterload, observed during high levels of spinal anesthesia. Systemic vascular resistance decreases only modestly, however, about 15% in normal individuals even in the presence of total preganglionic sympathetic denervation. This is because considerable arterial and arteriolar smooth muscle tone is retained following sympathetic denervation. Vasodilation is not maximal. Because systemic vascular resistance decreases only about 15% during total sympathetic denervation during spinal anesthesia, mean arterial pressure decreases only about 15% if cardiac output remains unchanged. Modest degrees of hypotension during spinal anesthesia can be ascribed to decreases in afterload. Severe degrees of hypertension cannot be due to this cause. Severe hypotension is due to decreases in cardiac output.

Whether cardiac output decreases or remains unchanged during spinal anesthesia depends upon what is happening in the simultaneously sympathetically denervated venous side of the circulation. Sympathetically denervated veins can, unlike arteries and arterioles, vasodilate.maximally. Whether they do so depends upon intraluminal hydrostatic pressure. If hydrostatic pressure remains low, there is little if any venodilation. If hydrostatic pressure increases, denervated veins dilate. Maximal dilation occurs in denervated veins when intraluminal pressures reach approximately 15 cmH_2O. Whether a pressure of 15 cmH_2O is reached depends principally on gravity. If denervated veins are 15 cm below the level of the right atrium, intraluminal pressure will be about 15 cmH_2O. The veins then dilate maximally. If only 6 cm below the level of the right atrium, denervated veins dilate, but not maximally.

The significance of venodilation during spinal anesthesia lies in the fact that the degree of venodilation determines venous return to the heart, i.e. pre-load, and, thus, cardiac output. Since position of the patient during spinal anesthesia determines the degree of venodilation, position is the critical determinant of pre-load. In the slight head-down position, venodilation is so minimal that pre-load and cardiac output remain unchanged. When cardiac output remains normal, mean arterial pressure decreases only about 15% due to the decrease in afterload. In the head-up position maximal peripheral venodilation occurs, and preload and cardiac output decrease. As cardiac output decreases, so, too, does mean arterial pressure. How much mean arterial pressure decreases depends upon the angle of the head-up position. Severe arterial hypotension during spinal anesthesia in normovolemic patients is due primarily to decreases in cardiac output secondary to decreases in pre-load following peripheral pooling of blood in the denervated venous circulation. In hypovolemic patients severe arterial can also occur, even with relatively limited degrees of sympathetic denervation, because pre-load may already be compromised and because what pre-load there is is dependent upon sympathetic venoconstriction.

Maintenance of adequate pre-load and adequate cardiac output and arterial perfusing pressure during spinal anesthesia depends upon avoidance of spinal anesthesia in the presence of hypovolemia and upon the judicious use of the head-down position for management or prevention of hypotension. The head-up position should be used for control of spread of hyperbaric or hypobaric local anesthetic solutions within the subarachnoid space. But if severe hypotension develops, the modest head-down position must be unhesitatingly and immediately used. Steep head-down position is unnecessary and may be counterproductive since the increase in internal jugular venous pressure associated with the steep head-down position decreases cerebral perfusing pressure. The level of anesthesia may rise, perhaps to embarrassingly high levels, when the head-down position is used to maintain blood pressure, but better unnecessarily high levels of anesthesia than cardiac arrest. It is unlikely that use of the head-down position for correction of arterial hypotension will result in impairment of respiration due to paralysis of the phrenic nerves. The same factors that give rise to a zone of differential sympathetic blockade also result in a zone of differential somatic motor blockade during spinal anesthesia. The level of somatic motor blockade averages two spinal segments below the level of sensory denervation. Mid-cervical levels of sensory anesthesia are therefore characteristically associated with no changes in diaphragmatic function. Even if apnea were to occur, this, in an era of ubiquitous use of neuromuscular relaxants, represents no major problem. The absence of spontaneous ventilation can be readily managed. Inadequate cardiac output cannot.

Venous return and cardiac output can also be maintained at adequate, if not at normal, levels during spinal anesthesia by the rapid intravenous infusion of large volumes of electrolyte solutions. This increases arterial pressure. It does so only at some physiologic cost in normovolemic patients. Of special concern is the effect of the rapid intravenous infusion of large volumes of crystalloid solutions in normovolemic patients on the balance between myocardial oxygen demands and myocardial oxygen supply. The hemodilution associated with the rapid intravenous infusion of large volumes of electrolyte solutions decreases the oxygen carrying capacity of arterial blood. This, in turn, means that at a given coronary perfusing pressure the rate at which oxygen is delivered to the myocardium does not increase in proportion to the increase in coronary blood flow. The decrease in rate of oxygen delivery occurs, however, at a time when myocardial oxygen demands are increased secondary to increases in pre-load and cardiac output. This may be of concern in patients with coronary arterial disease. Furthermore, the increase in pre-load associated with infusion of large volumes of electrolyte solutions increases ventricular end diastolic filling pressure. This, in turn, decreases subendocardial blood flow. To decrease subendocardial blood flow in the presence of a decrease in coronary perfusing pressure (arterial hypotension, plus increased end diastolic ventricular pressure) at a time when myocardial work load (increased pre-load) is increased but oxygen supply is not increased in parallel (because of hemodilution) may not represent an entirely satisfactory physiologic situation, especially in patients with coronary arterial disease. Blood pressure increases following the rapid infusion of large volumes of crystalloid solutions in normovolemic patients during spinal anesthesia, but blood pressure alone is a poor index of the adequacy of myocardial oxygenation. Reliance upon internal autotransfusion by use of the head-down position is a more physiologic approach. Use of large volumes of electrolyte solutions for restoration of blood pressure in normovolemic patients during spinal anesthesia also significantly increases the incidence of postoperative urinary retention requiring catheterization of the bladder. This, in turn, increases the risk of lower urinary tract infection.

Vasopressors, though frequently used for management of hypotension during spinal anesthesia in the past, are today relied upon infrequently because of the adverse effects on myocardial oxygenation with which they may be associated. Alpha-adrenergic agonists increase arterial pressure by increasing afterload. Decreases in afterload are, however, not the cause of hypotension during spinal anesthesia of a magnitude great enough to warrant treatment. The increase in afterload produced by alpha-adrenergic agonists may, furthermore, increase myocardial work and myocardial oxygen requirements more than they increase myocardial oxygen supply secondary to the increase in mean aortic pressure. Vasopressors that increase blood pressure by increasing myocardial contractility are also of limited use during spinal anesthesia. Hypotension severe enough to require pharmacologic intervention is due to decreases in pre-load, not to impaired myocardial contraction. Positive inotropic vasopressors also increased myocardal work and oxygen demands. Increasing contractility of "empty" ventricles during spinal anesthesia is not physiologically rational. Nor is use of vasopressors that increase blood pressure by increasing heart rate useful. The tachycardia they produce increases myocardial oxygen demands substantially more than they increase myocardial oxygen supply, especially since positive chronotropic vasopressors increase mean aortic pressure and coronary perfusing pressure only slightly. The ideal vasopressors for management of hypotension during spinal anesthesia would be those that have no effect except for production of venoconstriction. Such vasopressors would restore blood pressure by elimination of decreases in pre-load without adversely affecting other determinants of the ratio between myocardial oxygen demand and supply. Such selective vasopressors do not exist. Perhaps the best vasopressors to use, if hypotension is severe enough to require pharmacologic intervention because the head-down position has not been effective, are those such as ephedrine and mephentermine (Wyamine). They produce at least some venoconstriction while producing only relatively slight effects on afterload, heart rate, and myocardial contractility.

Concepts of how hypotension should be treated during spinal anesthesia have changed in tandem with concepts of when hypotension should be treated. Moderate levels of arterial hypotension during

spinal anesthesia are today no longer regarded as being deleterious.
Critical to this change in attitude toward hypotension has been
increased awareness of what changes in arterial pressure mean in terms
of myocardial oxygenation during spinal anesthesia. The relationships
between blood pressure, coronary blood flow and myocardial oxygenation
were first quantitated many years ago by Eckenhoff and his associates
(2). In dogs given spinal anesthesia, Eckenhoff, et al. found that
while mean arterial presure decreased an average of 37%, coronary blood
flow, a major determinant of myocardial oxygen supply, decreased 29%.
The decrease in coronary blood was also accompanied by a 65% decrease
in left ventricular work. The left ventricle was hyperperfused:
myocardial oxygen demands decreased more than myocardial oxygen
supply. Hackel and his associates (3) found similar responses during
spinal anesthesia in normal volunteers. Total preganglionic
sympathetic denervation produced by high thoracic levels of spinal
anesthesia decreased mean arterial pressure 48%. The hypotension was
associated with parallel decreases in both coronary blood flow (52%)
and left ventricular work (54%). In their subjects the myocardium was
not hyperperfused during spinal anesthesia, as it was in the dogs
studied by Eckenhoff, et al., but during hypotension the ratio between
myocardial oxygen demands and myocardial oxygen supply remained,
nevertheless, unchanged from pre-anesthetic control levels because
oxygen demands and supply decreased in parallel. Myocardial ischemia
did not occur despite hypotension of a magnitude great enough to
decrease coronary blood flow. High spinal anesthesia in monkeys is
associated with similar changes (4).

Spinal anesthesia decreases myocardial oxygen requirements in three
ways. First, the bradycardia that develops during the sympathetic
denervation associated with high spinal anesthesia decreases myocardial
work. Second, the decrease in afterload resulting from peripheral
arterial and arteriolar vasodilation decreases the amount of work the
left ventricle uses to eject a given amount of blood. And, third, the
decrease in preload, i.e. cardiac output, decreases the amount of work
expended over a given time.

Awareness that the ratio between myocardial oxygen requirements and
myocardial oxygen supply remains unaltered during moderate degrees of
hypotension during spinal anesthesia has led to realization that

moderate hypotension can and indeed should be tolerated since myocardial oxygenation, not arterial blood pressure, is our primary consideration. Whether the relationships between pressure, coronary flow and myocardial oxygen requirements observed in normal subjects during spinal anesthesia also apply to patients with coronary arterial disease has not been studied. However, cardiovascular responses to nitroglycerin and nitroprusside are remarkably similar to the cardiovascular responses to high spinal anesthesia. Nitroglycerin and nitroprusside are widely used in coronary care units to improve myocardial oxygenation. They are effective because they decrease pre-load and afterload. So, too, does spinal anesthesia. It is reasonable to apply the principles of the medical management of patients with coronary arterial disease to the anesthetic management of patients with possible or even demonstrable coronary arterial disease. For this reason coronary arterial disease is today no longer regarded as the contraindication to spinal anesthesia, especially low spinal anesthesia that it was in the past. Indeed, coronary arterial disease may actually be an indication for spinal anesthesia because of its salutary effects on the balance between myocardial oxygen supply and demand and because it has no effects on ventricular contractility.

Though maintenance of myocardial oxygenation means that moderate hypotension during spinal anesthesia need not, and perhaps should not, be treated, when aortic perfusing pressure decreases too far, coronary blood flow and myocardial oxygen supply decrease to the point where they are no longer adequate to maintain myocardial oxygenation even though myocardial oxygen demands are decreased. The critical level at which arterial pressure is no longer sufficient for maintenance of adequate myocardial oxygenation in the presence of simultaneous decreases in heart rate and in pre- and afterload during spinal anesthesia remains to be quantitated in normal subjects and in patients with coronary arterial disease. As a practical guide, mean arterial presures more than approximately 33% below normal resting values during spinal anesthesia can be regarded an indication for initiation of corrective measures. The first and most important corrective measure is, as discussed above, restoration of arterial pressure by use of the slight head-down position to increase pre-load and, thus, cardiac output. If this is not fully effective, then volume loading with

moderate amounts of crystalloid solutions and/or use of select
vasopressors should be employed.

REFERENCES

1. Space prohibits encyclopedic citation of the vast literature
   necessary to substantiate statements made and opinions expressed in
   this brief review. Instead, only 3 articles are cited and the
   reader is referred to the detailed discussions and extensive
   bibliography available in Chapters I and II of Greene, N.M.,
   Physiology of Spinal Anesthesia, 3rd Edition, Williams and Wilkins,
   Baltimore, 1981.
2. Eckenhoff JE, Hafkenschiel JH, Foltz EL et al. Influence of
   hypotension on coronary blood flow, cardiac work, and cardiac
   efficiency. Am J Physiol 1948;152:545-53.
3. Flackel DB, Sancetta SM, Kleinerman J. Effect of hypotension due to
   spinal anesthesia on coronary blood flow and myocardial metabolism
   in man. Circulation 1956;13:92-7.
4. Sivarajan M, Amory DW, Lindbloom LE et al. Systemic and regional
   blood flow changes during spinal anesthesia in Rhesus monkeys.
   Anesthesiology 1975;43:78-88.

CURRENT CONCEPTS AND PERSPECTIVES IN EPIDURAL ANAESTHESIA

PHILIP R. BROMAGE

You cannot make something work until you understand how it works. Epidural anesthesia has been with us since the turn of the century, but it is only in the last twenty-five years or so that the tools have become available to help us understand and exploit its mechanisms of action. We have come a long way in that time, and the most rapid advances have taken place in the past 5 years.

Site of Action

In 1885, Leonard Corning proposed the idea of medicating the spinal cord by injecting drugs close to it.[1] During the years that followed, this notion was dismissed as absurd, and the cord was not thought to be involved in subarachnoid or epidural blockade. Before 1950, the concepts of epidural analgesia were uncomplicated and straightforward. The dura mater was thought to be impermeable to local anesthetic. Epidural blockade was simply a matter of physical spread of local anesthetic in the extradural space, with outward passage through the intervertebral foramina to create a multiple, bilateral paravertebral block of the mixed spinal nerves beyond their dural cuffs, and just possibly by diffusion into the dorsal root ganglia as suggested by the predominantly sensory type of blockade. Since the dura was impermeable, local anesthetic could never reach intracranial structures, even in massive doses, and of course, the spinal cord would not be affected either.[2,3] All these assumptions and their clinical corollaries are now known to be partially or completely

false. Autoradiography and tissue assays have shown us that
the meninges are permeable to local anesthetics as well as to
narcotics of similar physicochemical characteristics, in
fact, passage from the extradural space into the CSF is so
rapid that the dura mater behaves almost as if it were not
there.[4,5,6,7] Intracranial structures can be involved (and
often are when epidural morphine is administered). And
finally, passage into the spinal roots and spinal cord always
occurs, with the cord as a primary site of sensory modulation.
Clinical radiographic studies have demonstrated that physical
spread of solutions in the epidural space does not coincide
with the dermatome level of segmental sensory blockade, and
the latter extends several segments beyond the limits of
radiographic spread.[8]

Neural tissue, CSF, blood vessels and fat all compete
for their share of local anesthetic or narcotic uptake from
the epidural space (Figure 1). The CSF scores heavily in
this scramble and CSF concentrations rise steeply. Drug
concentrations in the small volume of CSF are several orders
of magnitude higher than in the large pool represented by the
circulating blood volume. Concentrations in the fat depots
of the epidural space reflect the lipid solubility, protein-
binding and duration of the injected agents, and the epidural
fat seems to act as a reservoir for gradual release into the
adjacent subarachnoid space.[9] Epinephrine in concentrations
of 1/400,000 - 1/200,000 slows vascular absorption and sways
the competition for uptake in favor of CSF and neuraxial
tissues, prolonging and intensifying the quality of blockade.
However, the idea that epinephrine works solely through its
vascular effects is probably incorrect. Sensation is modulated
by a number of aminergic pathways within the brain and
spinal cord, and norepinephrine or epinephrine alone in the
epidural space produce a mild degree of segmental hypalgesia.[10,]

Now that the cord is seen as the ultimate target for
epidural analgesia, the mechanism of action of various drugs
has begun to take on a rational pattern. We understand how
epidural narcotics can penetrate to reach opiate receptors in

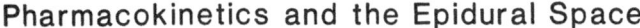

Pharmacokinetics and the Epidural Space

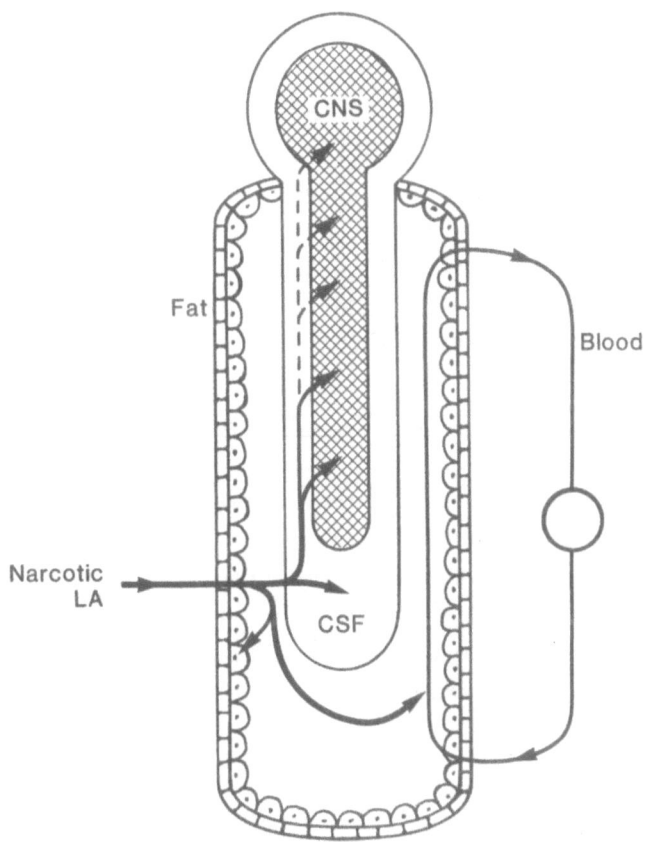

Figure 1: Pharmacokinetics and the epidural space.

Epidural narcotics and local anesthetics (LA) distribute
between epidural fat, cerebrospinal fluid (CSF), and
epidural blood vessels. The dura mater is a very
permeable barrier. Local anesthetics and narcotics
distribute between the CSF and the neuraxis according
to their lipid solubility: poorly lipid soluble agents
(such as morphine) spread rostrally in the CSF to reach
intracranial structures.

laminae 1 and 2 of the dorsal horn, thus producing intense
segmental antinociception. We can appreciate why we see
hyperreflexia in the legs after thoraco-cervical blocks, and
why upgoing toes are more apparent when we use a highly
lipid-soluble agent, such as etidocaine, that can penetrate
deeply to block the descending pyramidal pathways.[12a]

Measurements of vascular uptake from the epidural space
and placental transfer to the fetus at term pregnancy have
rationalized epidural analgesia in obstetrics. The factors
that reduce fetal uptake are well appreciated and techniques
can be standardized to ensure that the mother obtains the
greatest possible comfort with the least transfer of depressant
drugs to the uteroplacental unit.[12b]

PHYSIOLOGICAL EFFECTS OF EPIDURAL BLOCKADE

Clinical practice has been slow to catch up with advances
in the physiology of epidural blockade, and so it may be
useful to review some of the more important physiological
consequences of epidural blockade, since the "normal" reflex
physiological responses to surgery and trauma are often
inappropriate in a therapeutic setting. The major factors
that concern us are:

Sympathetic Blockade

1.   Hemodynamic Changes

Epidural local anesthetics produce blockade of sympathetic
efferents to a segmental level that corresponds precisely
with the level of skin analgesia. This causes segmental .
vasodilatation, with increased venous capacitance and increased
peripheral limb flow. Blockade above T_6 prevents vasoconstriction within the splanchnic bed, but then the splanchnic blood
flow becomes pressure dependent. Blockade extending above T_5
involves the cardiac inotropic and chronotropic fibres, with
a resulting fall in force and rate of ventricular contraction.
Some of these changes may be very beneficial during and after

major vascular surgery, when sympathetic blockade increases
graft flow and prevents reactive arterial hypertension. On
the other hand, the cardiovascular changes must be kept
within moderate and functional bounds, and this can be done
by using judicious combinations of crystalloid volume expansion
with vasopressor replacement therapy. That is to say, enough
vasopressor infusion is given to replace the small resting
output that has been suppressed by the action of the high
sympathetic blockade, and this usually implies a low concentration of dopamine or norephinephrine to provide the equivalent
of about 1 - 5 micrograms of norephinephrine per minute.

Epidural narcotics do not cause blockade of sympathetic
efferent pathways, and so these agents can be used to provide
pain relief alone, without any desirable or undesirable
effects on cardiovascular dynamics.[13] Thus, a fairly wide
range of therapeutic options exist with local anesthetics
alone or epidural narcotics alone, or with combinations of
the two (see Table 1).

TABLE 1

ATTRIBUTES OF EPIDURAL LOCAL ANESTHETICS vs EPIDURAL NARCOTICS

SEGMENTAL EFFECTS	LA	NARCOTIC
Pain	+	+
Proprioception	+	−
Vasomotor	+	−
Motor	+	−

2.   Metabolic Responses to Stress and Trauma

Splanchnic stimulation and outpouring of catecholamines
leads to splanchnic vasoconstriction, fall of visceral blood
flow and mobilization of metabolic substrates. Blood sugar
and cortisol rise and remain elevated for many hours postoperatively,[14] and nitrogen losses increase.[15] All these
changes are prevented by complete afferent blockade. However,
complete blockade of hypothalaminc stimulation is almost

impossible to achieve in upper abdominal and thoracic surgery, when normal hormonal responses (activated through the hypothalamic-pituitary axis) persist due to unblocked vagal and phrenic afferent stimuli, in spite of high segmental blockade. Thus, the hope of complete protection from hormonal responses to stress is only realized in operations on the lower parts of the body and trunk.

Afferent Blockade

Nature seeks to protect and immobilize an injured part. Broken ribs and knife wounds of the belly are followed by shallow grunting respiration and an inability to take deep breaths and to cough effectively. Injured backs are held stiffly, and wounded knees are locked in partial flexion. Some of these protective postures are appropriate, but after upper abdominal or thoracic surgery or total knee replacement, local muscle spasm may be harmful. The chest must move, and the patient must be able to cough up his bronchial secretions. Interruption of the afferent side of the reflex arc permits the patient to take deep breaths and to cough effectively. On the other hand, excessive freedom of back movement after a laminectomy may be frankly harmful in an area that is better left at rest. Given proper technical management, both epidural local anesthetics and epidural narcotics can be of great respiratory benefit after laparotomy or thoracotomy, and either type of drug can restore a mechanical respiratory deficit of 70% to one of 30% below preoperative control values on the day of operation.[16]

If the afferent side of the reflex arc alone could be broken in all operative situations, we would see perfect analgesia with no autonomic or motor side effects. Unfortunately, pure deafferentation is difficult to achieve, and pain relief with epidural local anesthetics is inevitably accompanied by vasomotor block and some degree of motor weakness within the segmental area of blockade. The epidural narcotics afford an escape from these unwanted aspects of neural blockade, since narcotic spinal blockade is a relatively pure event and free of sympathetic effects. However, as we shall see, the epidural narcotics have their own problems, and therapeutic skill lies in finding a proper balance among the limited analgesic options that are available.

Epidural Narcotics

In this review of perspectives, epidural narcotics require special consideration, not so much for what they do of themselves, as for what they represent, standing as they do at the threshold between the old pharmacology of intra-spinal local anesthetics and the new era of neuraxial pharmacology and sensory modulation within the spinal cord.

Historically, the intraspinal narcotics were a first attempt to apply the basic neuraxial pharmacology of antino-ciception in the clinical arena, as an extension of Corning's idea of nearly one hundred years ago, that medication of the spinal cord might be possible by injecting drugs in close proximity to it.[1] In the early 1970s, narcotics were shown to act upon opiate receptors in Rexed's laminae 1 and 2 of the dorsal horn.[17] Although opiate receptors can be found along the length of axons, their numbers are few and narcotics do not produce axonal blockade. Their greatest density is to be found at pre- and post-synaptic sites in the small cell networks of laminae 1 and 2, in the sensory nucleus of the trigeminal nerve (a cranial extension of the dorsal horn), in the periaqueductal gray matter, and in many of the visceral nuclei lying just under the ependymal floor of the 4th ventricle. In the dorsal horn narcotic action is almost purely antinociceptive, and there is no involvement of sympathetic or motor functions. Herein lies the possibility of achieving segmental pain blockade, without the cost of vasomotor and motor blockade that is the price to be paid for axonal block with local anesthetics.

Early clinical reports of intrathecal and epidural morphine were enthusiastic and full of promise. Intense segmental analgesia of extremely long duration was indeed obtained with very small doses of morphine and without respiratory depression.[18,19] A flurry of laboratory and clinical studies followed, and while these investigations confirmed the great analgesic power of the new techniques, they also revealed a high incidence of serious side effects. It was soon apparent that the segmental nature of the spinal narcotics was not reliable, but depended on the drug used. While the lipid-soluble agents such as fentanyl, meperidine, methadone and hydromophone did seem to provide a relatively stable segmental area of analgesia,[13] morphine with its low lipid solubility, tended to migrate rostrally, and 10 mg in the epidural space spread upwards to involve lower trigeminal territory by the 7th hour.[20] Cephalad migration proceeded further and faster to reach the 5th nerve by the 5th hour if epinephrine 1/200,000 was added to the morphine.[21] Along with this rostral spread went nonsegmental pruritus, prolonged urinary retention and increased bladder compliance.[22,23] and marked depression of respiratory sensitivity to CO_2 between the 6th and 12th hours.[24]

In the meantime, other intraspinal agents were being investigated, and drugs acting on peptide and aminergic pathways were found to modulate pain sensation.[10] Future work will probably be directed towards nociceptive modulation through neurotransmitters or transmitter-analogues that have little or no intrinsic narcotic properties at opiate-receptor sites. We shall probably see opiates and neuromodulators used in combination in order to obtain the best suppression of nociception with least side effects, by actions at multiple sites and on different interlocking modulatory systems.

CLINICAL APPLICATIONS: RATIONALE AND APOLOGIA FOR EPIDURAL BLOCKADE

In all the applications of epidural analgesia, the apologia for its use rests upon three capabilities:
1. Segmental relief of pain

2.   Preservation of respiratory and motor function
     through blockade of the afferent side of the
     reflex arc and suppression of reflex muscle spasm
3.   Segmental sympathetic afferent blockade with:
     a.   segmental vasodilatation and increased peripheral
          limb blood flow
     b.   suppression of adrenal medullary response to
          stress
     c.   suppression of adrenal cortical response to
          stress BUT ONLY IF AFFERENT BLOCKADE IS COMPLETE

Of these three attributes, relief of pain is constant to
all clinical applications; the other two have variable
indications. And yet, relief of pain alone does not constitute
a solid reason for using epidural analgesia. Indeed, one may
argue, does pain really matter? Pain of itself can be endured,
and has been through the millenia. Pain is part of mans'
estate, and of itself, it is not life threatening. It is not
pain, but the body's protective reactions to pain - the
muscle spasm and the sympathetic responses, that threaten
life and limb. Pain by itself can be completely relieved and
life supported by prolonged general anesthesia, neuromuscular
blockade and artificial ventilation, for days on end if
necessary. Rather, it is the other two attributes, preservation
of motor function and avoidance of reflex vasoconstriction
that make epidural analgesia unique as a therapeutic modality.
Unless these latter attributes are exploited in an appropriate
fashion, there is little logic in touting epidural blockade
as a rational alternative or as a complement to modern general
anesthesia.

Surgery and Trauma

There is no sense in administering a superb epidural
anesthetic with the long-acting agents bupivacaine or etidocaine,
if the operation is relatively short, and if the patient is
left to lie in the recovery room at great expense, immobile
and totally motor-blocked from the xiphisterum down for the

160

next four hours (see Figure 2).

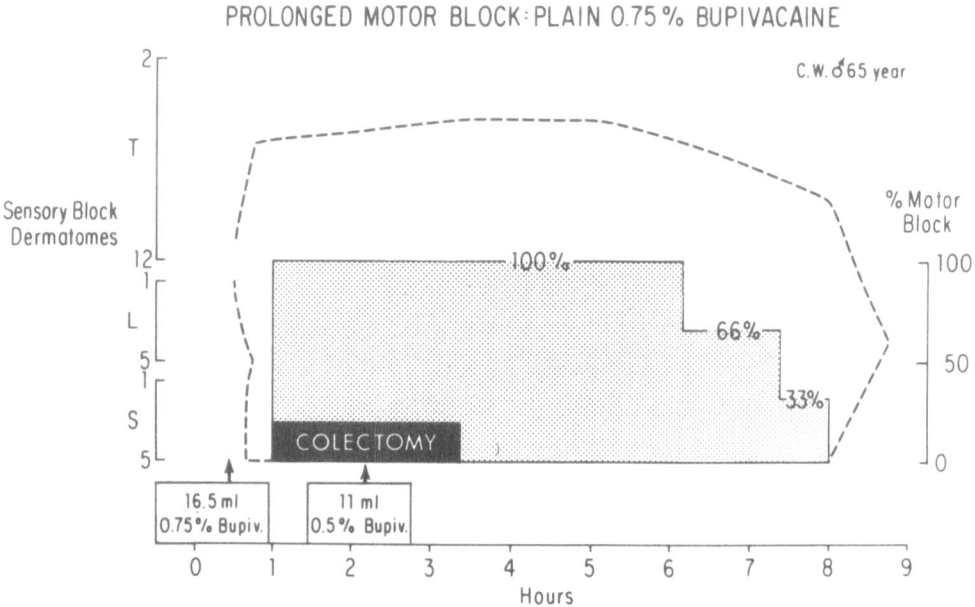

PROLONGED MOTOR BLOCK: PLAIN 0.75% BUPIVACAINE

Figure 2: Example of inappropriate functional use of epidural
analgesia.

This 65 year old man lay immobile for 3 hours after major
surgery. Choice of a shorter acting local anesthetic
would have permitted active leg exercises during that period

He will be pain-free, certainly, and the legs will be
vasodilated and total blood flow to the legs may be increased.
But the calf muscle-pump will be inactivated and venous flow
through the deep veins will depend entirely in complex
hemodynamic constraints that tend to redistribute blood flow
from muscle into skin,[25] and the risk of deep-vein thrombosis
in the calf will be increased rather than decreased.

Obstetrics

The functional benefits of epidural analgesia are more obvious in obstetrics than in surgery. With proper technique, maternal doses are relatively small, and only miniscule amounts of potentially depressant local anesthetic cross the placenta to reach the baby. Pain and anxiety can be relieved while the forces of labour are well sustained. Tone can be maintained in the pelvic floor to aid normal rotation of the fetal head, and the abdominal expulsive forces can be kept almost fully intact.

In this field, mixtures of epidural local anesthetics and lipid-soluble narcotics are still in an exploratory stage. Clinical evidence to date suggests that weak concentrations of bupivacaine (such as the 0.125% solution) with small amounts of fat-soluble narcotic, such as fentanyl in 50 - 60 ug doses may represent an important practical advance in terms of maximizing pain-relief and function at least cost from drug-induced depression.[26]

Chronic Pain

Epidural and subarachnoid narcotics have supplanted local anesthetics for the palliative management of malignant pain. Effective pain relief can be maintained for weeks or months by home administration through exterior epidural catheters or by surgically implanted reservoirs that can be refilled percutaneously. Small doses of epidural morphine in the range of 4 - 5 mg seem to be effective in these cases.

RISK AND COST/BENEFIT RATIOS

Pain relief is always bought at a cost. The risk may be high and life threatening if an overdose of narcotic causes dangerous respiratory depression. The risk may be one of morbidity if the cough reflex is excessively depressed and bronchial secretions accumulate, or it may be just a nuisance if a narcotic causes nausea and depressed bowel function.

How does epidural analgesia rank in this sort of risk-analysis? Well enough, if we look at the superb quality and segmental nature and duration of analgesia that can be obtained, but no so well if we count the risks and costs carefully. We are constantly haunted by the fear of neural damage from trauma, infection, hematoma or chemical irritation, remote though these risks may be. While these risks are extremely small numerically, qualitatively they are horrendous, and their rare visitation may bring ruin to a victim's life. This fear lingers for as long as epidural pain relief is maintained. In the postoperative period, the most carefully metered epidural infusions cannot guarantee that the calculated dose will match the individual's requirements precisely. We never know whether the segmental level from an infusion may creep too high in the small morning hours, with a resulting fall in blood pressure, and perhaps clotting of a grafted vessel from the reduced perfusion pressure. Similarily, infusions of epidural narcotics may spread rostrally to cause apnoeic spells which may not be noted until too late, if the victim is asleep in the comfort of a single-bedded room, with the door closed.

Not one of our recent advances in pain management has cut the ancient knot binding the risk of respiratory depression to relief from pain, and least of all the epidural narcotics.[11,24,27,28,29] And so we come back to where we were before these new techniques evolved. The sick and suffering need surveillance and the patient receiving epidural analgesia, by local anesthetics or by narcotics, needs it most emphatically if he is to escape the growing list of apnoeic statistics arising from these powerful techniques.

What does appropriate surveillance cost, and is it worth the price?

In these days of cost-conciousness and accountability, we must ask this practical question, and we must answer it, for if we do not, our hospital administrators and our political masters will do it for us, and we may find that pain-relief

comes low on the list of priorities for scarce financial
resources.

The answer to this question of costs is easy to obtain
in the North American context, and it is thought-provoking.
Close surveillance in an intensive-care milieu costs about
four times as much as a private hospital room, and approximately
one thousand dollars for 24 hours. No one can pretend that a
private room with the door closed is anything but a potential
death trap in the presence of respiratory depression. And
so, if we are to exploit the most elegant forms of analgesia
that exists today, the price of safety is very high.

Would you pay such a price for the extra comfort for so
short a while, or would you exercise prudent fortitude, and
endure with the help of such analgesia as is afforded by
traditional narcotic prescriptions?

For the majority of us, the answer is clear. We would
not waste our money in so craven a fashion, unless there were
some other very good reason - unless the costly technique
brought some other unique benefit that might contribute to a
safe and rapid recovery. And here we might be persuaded by
the functional benefits of epidural analgesia. But the
functional restoration bestowed by epidural analgesia is
often wasted on the young and fit. They seldom need it.
They will survive most routine surgical assaults under routine
general anesthesia, and make an uncomplicated recovery, in
spite of the functional deficits that postoperative pain
causes. It is the old and infirm, and patients with one or
more failing vital systems that need the immediate functional
recovery that epidural analgesia can provide. Thus, it is
not the pain itself, but the functional disturbances arising
from the pain that makes the cost worthwhile.

And so, we come to a second question: how can we reduce
the high cost without losing either efficacy or safety? How
can we trim the vast expense of modern intensive care to fit
the relatively simple needs of respiratory surveillance
during prolonged postoperative analgesia? There is a movement
to reconsider some sort of multibedded open ward with a few

well-trained and dedicated nurses in charge. Florence Nightingale used this principle at Scutari in 1854, and the 30-bedded Victorian Ward survived for many years as one of the safest places in which to be ill. The modern intensive care unit is really just an extension of the principle of the Victorian Ward, but at a very expensive level of high technology.

Somewhere between the unsafe luxury of the single room and the expensive safety of the intensive care unit, there is a compromise to be made, and a return to the concept of the Victorian Ward fits this need as a staging post between the recovery area and the private room. Such a compromise could be elastic, as a Pain Ward within the range of 8 to 30 beds, staffed by perhaps 3 nurses under the direction of an anesthesiologist, and possibly supplemented by apnoea alarms. A unit of this sort could be cost-effective, and it could come close to the ideal of combining safety with effective control of pain and maximum restoration of function. The future survival of epidural analgesia as a practical technique (or indeed any other mode of effective pain control) will depend upon the adoption of this type of economical facility where a successful marriage can be made between the benefits of effective pain control, and the safe containment of the accompanying risks. In achieving this marriage, we shall have to acknowledge the foresight of old lessons and past ideas that have almost been forgotten. Leonard Corning's notion of medicating the spinal cord, and Florence Nightingale's organizational genius in the Crimea can point the way to effective control of pain and restoration of function in a safe but affordable fashion.

REFERENCES

1. Corning J L (1885) Spinal anaesthesia and local medication of the cord. N Y Med J 42:483
2. Dogliotti A M (1931) Anesthesia. S D Debour, Chicago p 537
3. Dawkins C J M (1945) Extradural spinal block. Proc Roy Soc Med 38:299
4. Bromage P R, Joyal A C and Binney J C (1963) Local anesthetic drugs: Penetration from the spinal extradural space into the neuraxis. Science 140:392-393
5. Moore R A, Bullingham R E, McQuay H J, Hand C W, Aspel J B, Allen M C and Thomas D (1982) Dural permeability to

narcotics: In vitro determination and application to
extradural administration. Brit J Anaes 54:1117-1128

6. Cousins M J, Mather C, Glynn C J (1979) Selective spinal
anesthesia. Lancet 1:1141-1142

7. Nordberg G, Hedner T, Mellstrand T and Dahlstrom B (1983)
Pharmacokinetic aspects of epidural morphine analgesia.
Anesthesiology 58:545-551

8. Schulte-Steinberg O and Rahlfs V W (1970) Caudal anaesthesia
in children and spread of 1 per cent lignocaine: A
statistical study. Brit J Anaesth 42:1093-1099

9. Tucker G T, and Mather L E (1980) Absorption and disposition
of local anesthetics: Pharmacokenetics. in Neural Blockade
in Clinical Management of Pain. J B Lippincot Company,
Phil. and Toronto pp 45-85

10. Yaksh T L and Ramana Reddy S V (1981) Studies in the
Primate on the analgetic effects associated with intrathecal
actions of opiates, a-Adrenergic agonists and baclofen.
Anesthesiology 54:451-467

11. Bromage P R, Camporesi E M, Durant P A and Nielsen C H
(1983) Influence of Epinephrine as as adjuvant to epidural
morphine. Anesthesiology 58:257-262

12a. Bromage P R, O'Beirn P and Dunford L A (1974b) Etidocaine:
A clinical evaluation for regional analgesia in surgery.
Canad Anaesth Soc J 21:523-534

12b. Bromage P R (1978) Table 12-3 Placental transfer of
local anesthetics in lumbar epidural and caudal blockade
during labor. in Epidural Analgesia. W B Saunders
Company, Phil., London and Toronto pp 536-537

13. Bromage P R, Camporesi E and Leslie J (1980) Epidural
narcotics in volunteers: sensitivity to pain and to carbon
dioxide. Pain 9:145-160

14. Bromage P R, Shibata H R and Willoughby H W (1971)
Influence of prolonged epidural blockade on blood sugar
and cortisol responses to operations upon the upper part
of abdomen and the thorax. Surg Gynecol Obstet
132:1051-1056

15. Brandt M R, Fernandes A, Mordhurst R et al (1978) Epidural
analgesia improves postoperative nitrogen balance. Brit
Med J i:1106-1108

16. Bromage P R, Camporesi E M, Chestnut D (1980) Epidural
narcotics for postoperative analgesia. Anesth & Analg
59:473-480

17. Calvillo O, Henry J L, Neuman R S (1974) Effects of morphine
and naloxone on dorsal horn neurones in the cat. Can J
Physiol Pharmacol 52:1207-1211

18. Wang J L, Nauss L A and Thomas J E (1979) Pain relief by
intrathecally applied morphine in man. Anesthesiology
50:149-151

19. Behar M, Olshwang D, Magora F and Davidson J T (1979)
Epidural morphine in treatment of pain. Lancet 1:527-528

20. Bromage P R, Camporesi E M, Durant P A C and Nielsen C H
(1982) Rostral spread of epidural morphine. Anesthesiology
56:431-436

21. Bromage P R, Camporesi E M, Durant P A and Nielsen C H
(1983) Influence of epinephrine as an adjuvant to epidural

morphine.   Anesthesiology 58:257-262
22. Bromage P R, Camporesi E M, Durant P A C and Nielsen C H
    (1982) Nonrespiratory side effects of epidural morphine.
    Anesth & Analg 61:490-495
23. Rawal N, Mollefors K, Axelsson K, Lingardh G and Widman B
    (1983) An experimental study of urodynamic effects of
    epidural morphine and of naloxone reversal.   Anesth &
    Analg 62:641-647
24. Camporesi E M, Nielsen C H, Bromage P R, Durant, P A C
    (1983) Ventilatory CO_2 sensitivity after intravenous and
    epidural morphine in volunteers. Anesth & Analg 62:633-640
25. Cousins M J and Wright C J (1971) Graft, muscle, skin blood
    flow after epidural block in vascular surgical procedures.
    Surg Gynecol Obstet 133:59-64
26. Justins D M, Houlton P G, Reynolds F (1982) Controlled
    trial of extradural fentanyl in labour.   Brit J Anaesth
    54:409-414
27. Doblar D D, Muldoon S M, Albrecht P H, Baskoff J, Watson R I
    (1981) Epidural morphine following epidural local anesthesia
    effect on ventilatory and airway occlusion pressure response
    to CO_2.   Anesthesiology 66:423-428
28. Kafer E R, Brown J T, Scott D, Findlay J W A, Butz R F,
    Teeple E and Ghia J N (1983) Biphasic Depression of
    Ventilatory Responses to CO_2 Following Epidural Morphine.
    Anesthesiology 58:418-427
29. Knill R L, Clement J L, Thompson W R (1981) Epidural morphine
    causes delayed and prolonged ventilatory depression.   Canad
    Anaesth Soc J 28:537-543

PHARMACOKINETICS IN SPINAL AND EPIDURAL ANAESTHESIA

A.G.L. BURM AND J.W. VAN KLEEF

1. INTRODUCTION

The processes that determine the fate of a local anaesthetic agent after its injection into the subarachnoid or epidural space are local disposition, systemic absorption and systemic disposition.[1] These processes are not independent, but for the ease of understanding they are usually considered separately. In this paper we will concentrate on local disposition and systemic absorption. For a review on the systemic disposition the reader is referred to the existing literature.[1,2] Some of the factors that affect the systemic absorption and disposition are dealt with in the chapter by Tucker on the effects of regional blood flow changes.

2. LOCAL DISPOSITION

The term local disposition includes both distribution of the agents into and out of the tissues at and near the site of injection and elimination of the agent from the site of injection and its surroundings. Elimination of local anaesthetics from the subarachnoid and epidural spaces and their surroundings occurs by vascular absorption and will therefore be considered separately.

Most of the ideas about local distribution are based on indirect evidence, and therefore remain theoretical. The events that determine the local distribution of a local anaesthetic agent are physical spread, diffusion, tissue binding and probably also vascular transport.

Physical spread of the local anaesthetic reflects bulk flow of the solution and depends mainly upon the volume of the injected solution, the speed or better the force of injection and the resistance to bulk flow, the volume of the space and finally gravity and the posture of the patient. For example, 5 ml of a local anaesthetic solution, injected into the subarachnoid space with a specified force, will spread further than 2 ml, injected with the same force.[3] Similarly 40 ml of a solution, injected into the epidural space might be expected to spread further than 20 ml.[4,7] This is not necessarily accompanied by a greater analgesic spread, especially not after epidural administration. Bromage [5] has demonstrated that the analgesic spread following epidural

administration of local anaesthetic solutions depends mainly
upon the mass of local anaesthetic and not so much upon the
volume that is injected. This suggests that other mechanisms
such as diffusion and perhaps vascular transport are more
important as determinant of local anaesthetic dispersion
after epidural administration. An increase in the speed of
injection may theoretically result in a more extensive spread
of the anaesthetic, but in practice the effect is probably
very small.[4,6,7] The effect of the volume of the space is
readily observed in practice: if the volume of the epidural
or subarachnoid space is reduced then a given volume of
anaesthetic results in much higher analgesia levels, which
are probably due to a more extensive physical spread of the
anaesthetic. This may be observed for example in pregnant
women at term and in patients with intra-abdominal tumors,
where the chronically increased intra-abdominal pressure and
the resulting chronic engorgement of the epidural veins and
rise in the extradural pressure cause a decrease in the
volume of the epidural space as well as the volume of cerebrospinal fluid.[8-10] Acute increases in intra-abdominal pressure or acute engorgement of epidural veins might increase
the spread within the epidural space but probably have little
effect on the dispersion within the subarachnoid space, since
in this situation the increased pressure will result in an
increase in cerebrospinal fluid pressure rather than a decrease in the volume of cerebrospinal fluid.[8]

The effects of gravity and the posture of the patient are
well recognized in spinal anaesthesia. For example when a
hyperbaric solution is injected into the subarachnoid space
of a patient who is sitting upright, then the bulk of local
anaesthetic will descend and disperse in the lumbosacral
area.[8] If the same solution is injected into a patient in the
head down position then the solution may ascend resulting in
a greater thoracic spread. Gravity may also promote downward
spread of the local anaesthetic solution within the epidural
space of a patient sitting upright compared to the spread in
a patient in the lateral position.[10,11]

After the local anaesthetic has been deposited and physi-
cally spread it finds its way to the sites of action in and
on the nerve membrane by diffusion. On its way to the axonal
membrane it may have to pass several diffusion barriers. The
driving force for the diffusion process is the concentration
gradient from the site of injection to the targets. Any
factor, that affects concentrations at any site between the
site of injection and the site of action has an impact on the
diffusion process and consequently on the amount of anaesthetic that ultimately reaches the sites of action and the rate
at which this occurs. These factors include vascular absorption at the site of injection or along the pathway to the
axons and binding to non-specific binding sites both extra-
neural and intraneural, such as proteins or fat tissues. Also
pH differences across membranes are important. Local anaesthetics exist in two forms in aquous solutions, namely the
uncharged free base form and the charged cationic form. Both
forms may diffuse in aquous solutions such as the cerebrospi-

nal fluid or other extracellular or intracellular media, but only the free base form can diffuse through lipid membranes. The ratio of the concentrations of the free drug and the charged cationic form depends upon the pKa of the drug and the pH of the medium. The higher the pKa and the lower the pH the less of the anaesthetic will be in the free base form. Therefore pH differences across membranes will alter the diffusion since they affect the concentration gradient of the free base form.

The impact of diffusion and non specific binding can readily be demonstrated when the onset and the duration of the block following epidural and subarachnoid injection of a local anaesthetic are considered. Both techniques have common major sites of action, namely the spinal nerves within the subarachnoid space and the (periphery of the) spinal cord. In addition blockade of paravertebral nerves may contribute to epidural anaesthesia.[11]

When a local anaesthetic is injected into the subarachnoid space it is diluted by mixing with the cerebrospinal fluid, but despite of this the initial concentrations in cerebrospinal fluid are relatively high.[12,13] Within the cerebrospinal fluid there are relatively few binding sites for local anaesthetics since the lipid content and the number of protein binding sites are limited. Therefore, immediately after the injection there will be a high concentration gradient, between the cerebrospinal fluid on the one hand and the individual axons in the nerves and the periphery of the cord on the other. This also applies to the free base form, despite a slight decrease in the CSF pH which is usually observed after injection of a local anaesthetic solution. Furthermore the spinal nerves lack epineurium and epineural sheath tissues which surround peripheral nerves. Therefore the number of diffusion barriers is limited. All factors, the high concentration gradient, the limited binding and the limited number of diffusion barriers promote the rapid diffusion to and through the axonal membrane and into the spinal cord, where sufficient concentrations will build up rapidly, which results in the rapid onset of blockade, which is observed clinically.

On the other hand, when a local anaesthetic is injected into the epidural space much of the dose may dissolve in the epidural fat tissue and only a fraction of the dose will be available for diffusion to the targets. In order to reach the cerebrospinal fluid the anaesthetic must pass the dura, either directly by passive diffusion or by active transport or diffusion through the arachnoid villi at the dural route sleeves.[1,11] The initial cerebrospinal fluid concentrations following epidural administration are relatively low compared to the concentrations after subarachnoid injection.[14,15] Centripetal spread from the paravertebral trunks through the subperineural and subpial spaces to the periphery of the spinal cord may also contribute to the block.[11] In any case the anaesthetic has to travel a longer distance and has to pass more diffusion barriers following epidural anaesthesia. These limiting factors probably contribute much to the slower onset of epidural anaesthesia, despite the much higher doses that are administered epidurally.

Binding and diffusion barriers not only have an impact on the onset of blockade and on the clinical potency of the agent, but also on the duration of action. By slow dissociation of the local anaesthetic from the binding sites the diffusion gradient towards the axons will be maintained and diffusion our of the nerve will be slowed. Diffusion barriers also restrict the outward diffusion. Both binding and diffusion barriers will therefore result in a prolongation of the block and this may contribute to the longer duration of an epidural block compared to a subarachnoid block.

Finally, local binding may also restrict vascular uptake.

3. SYSTEMIC ABSORPTION

Systemic absorption is more accessible for investigation compared to local distribution. Measurements of plasma or whole blood concentrations have revealed a lot of information on the absorption of local anaesthetics after various regional anaesthetic procedures and upon the factors that modify absorption in particular. However, a detailed interpretation of the plasma concentration curves is only possible if the data on the systemic disposition are available.[1,2] The plasma concentration curves obtained after epidural administration have shown that within a few minutes measurable concentrations are reached, which demonstrates that the absorption must start immediately or almost immediately after the administration.[2,16] The concentration then rises further until a peak is reached, usually 10 to 40 minutes after the administration (Fig. 1). Beyond this time the amount of drug that is removed from the blood exceeds the amount that is absorbed and consequently the blood level falls. From the slope of the terminal part of the plasma conentration curve the elimination half-life can be calculated, which is in the order of 3-7 hours for lidocaine and 7-10 hours for bupivacaine. If one compares this value with the average elimination half-life following intravenous administration which is 1.5-2.0 h for lidocaine and somewhat less than 3 hours for bupivacaine one may wonder why the half-lives are so much prolonged after epidural anaesthesia, since it seems unlikely that epidural anaesthesia by itself has such an impact on the steady state volume of distribution or clearance that this results in a nearly threefold increase in the half-life. The solution to this puzzle was given by investigations of Tucker and Mather, who determined the absorption kinetics after epidural anaesthesia, using the data on disposition kinetics obtained after intravenous administration of the same agents to the same volunteers. The results of their study showed that the absorption of local anaesthetics after epidural anaesthesia is a biphasic process.[2] The rapid absorption phase is characterized by a short half-life. For example, the values obtained by Tucker and Mather were in the order of 10-20 min for lidocaine and 20 minutes for bupivacaine. The slow

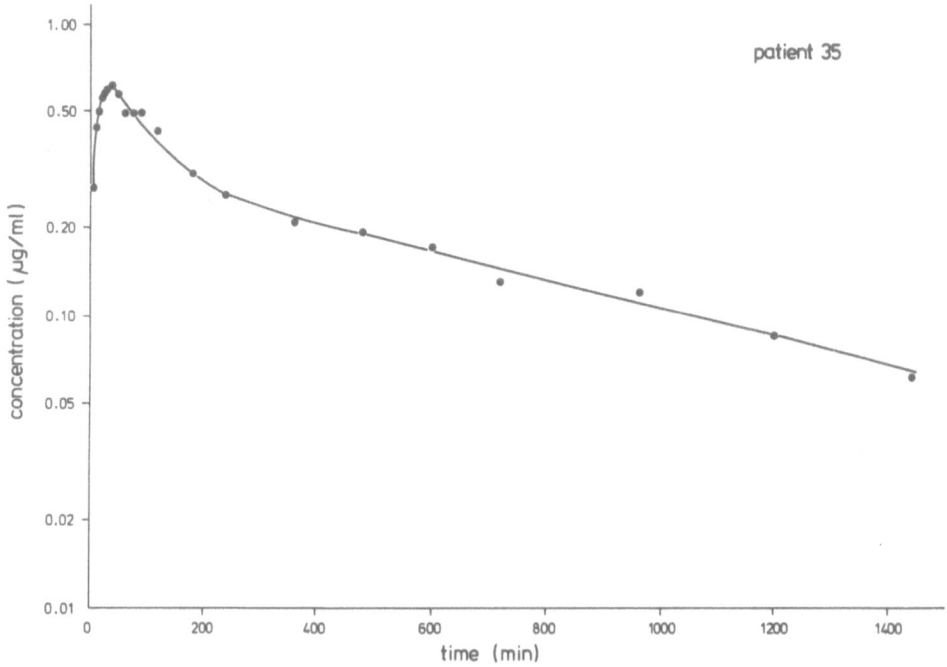

Fig 1. Typical plasma concentration curve, obtained after epidural administration of 150 mg bupivacaine.[16]

absorption phase is characterized by a long half-life which amounts 3-7 h for lidocaine and about 7 h for bupivacaine. The rapid absorption phase is reflected in the plasma concentration curve following epidural administration, as a short peak time, while the slow absorption phase is reflected in the long elimination half-life, which in this situation equals in fact the absorption half-life.

A typical curve obtained after subarachnoid administration of 15 mg bupivacaine is shown in Fig. 2. This curve differs in several respects from the curve obtained after epidural administration of bupivacaine (Fig. 1). This applies to both the peak time and the elimination half-life. The peak times obtained after subarachnoid administration of hyperbaric solutions of lidocaine and bupivacaine in our studies were on average about 1 hour,[17] which is considerably longer than the average peak times of 20-25 minutes, which have been obtained after epidural administration. The peak times which have been measured after subarachnoid administration of isobaric solutions of bupivacaine are even longer and averaged 90 min. The longer peak times observed after subarachnoid administration are associated with relatively low peak concentrations. The available data demonstrate that the normalized concentrations obtained after epidural anaesthesia are about 25-50 percent higher than the concentrations measured after subarachnoid

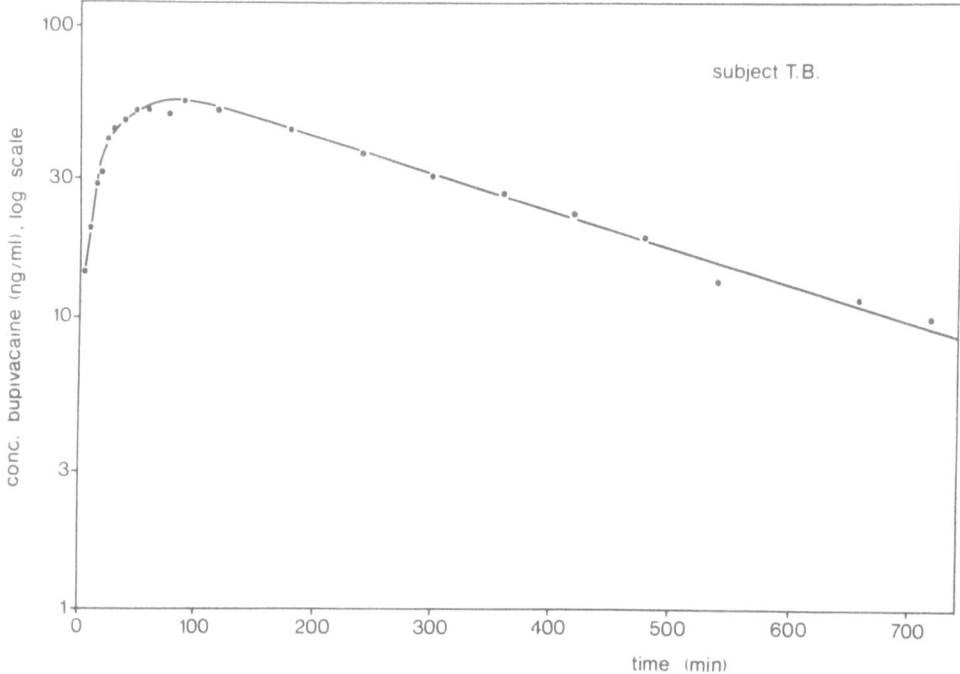

Fig 2.   Typical plasma concentration curve obtained after
subarachnoid administration of 15 mg bupivacaine.[17]

administration.

Both the increased peak times and the lower peak concentrations obtained after subarachnoid administration suggest
that the initial absorption rate is slower after subarachnoid
injection than after epidural injection.

The elimination half-lives determined after subarachnoid
administration averaged 2.0 h for lidocaine and about 3.5 h
for bupivacaine. A comparison of these values with the values
obtained after epidural administration of lidocaine and bupivacaine demonstrates that the elimination half-lives are
considerably longer after epidural injection. As mentioned
above the long half-life after epidural administration results from the slow absorption of a part of the dose. The
much shorter elimination half-lives obtained after subarachnoid administration, which are in fact close to the elimination half-lives determined after intravenous administration,
suggest that the slow absorption phase, associated with epidural administration, is lacking or is at least much less
predominant after subarachnoid administration. This has been
confirmed recently in monkeys.[18] Whether the absorption after
subarachnoid administration in man can be considered as a
biphasic process or not remains to be clarified and requires
investigations of the absorption kinetics.

References
1. Tucker GT, Mather LE. Absorption and disposition of local anesthetics. In: Neural Blockade, Ed. Cousins MJ, Bridenbaugh PO. 1980. J.B. Lippincott Co., pp 45-85, Philadelphia/Toronto.
2. Tucker GT, Mather LE. Clinical pharmacokinetics of local anesthetics. Clin Pharmacokinet. 4: 241-278, 1979.
3. Rieselbach RE, Di Chiro G, Freireich EJ, Rall D.P. Subarachnoid distribution of drugs after lumbar injection. N. Engl. J. Med. 267: 1273-1278, 1962.
4. Burn JM, Guyer PB, Langdon L. The spread of solutions injected into the epidural space. A study using epidurograms in patients with the lumbosciatic syndrome. Br. J. Anaesth. 45: 338-345, 1973.
5. Bromage, PR. Mechanism of action of extradural analgesia. Br. J. Anaesth. 47, Suppl.: 199-211, 1975.
6. Neigh JL, Kane PB, Smith TC. Effects of speed and direction of injection on the level and duration of spinal anesthesia. Anesth. Analg. 49: 912-918,1970.
7. Erdemir HA, Soper LE, Sweet RB. Studies of factors affecting peridural anesthesia. Anesth. Analg. 44: 400-404, 1965.
8. Greene NM. 1981. Physiology of spinal anesthesia, 3rd ed. Williams and Wilkins, Baltimore/London.
9. Barclay DL, Renegar OJ, Nelson EW. The influence of inferior vena cava compression on the level of spinal anesthesia. Am. J. Obstet. Gynecol. 101: 792-800, 1968.
10. Bromage PR. 1978. Epidural analgesia. W.B. Saunders Company, Philadelphia.
11. Bromage PR. Spread of analgesic solutions in the epidural space and their site of action: a statistical study. Br. J. Anaesth. 34: 161-178, 1962.
12. Mörch ET, Rosenberg MK, Truant AT. Lidocaine for spinal anaesthesia. Acta Anaesthesiol. Scand. 1: 105-115, 1957.
13. Meyer J, Nolte H. Liquorkonzentration von Bupivacaine nach subduraler Applikation. Regional-Anaesthesie 1: 38-40, 1978.
14. Lund PC, Covino BG. Distribution of local anesthetics in man following peridural anesthesia. J. Clin. Pharmacol 7: 324-329, 1967.
15. Wilkinson GR, Lund PC. Bupivacaine levels in plasma and cerebrospinal fluid following peridural administration. Anesthesiology 33: 482-486, 1970.
16. Van Kleef JW. 1981. A clinical evaluation of bupivacaine (Marcaine[R]) 0.5% versus 0.75%. Ph.D. Thesis, State University of Leiden.
17. Burm AG, Van Kleef JW, Gladines MP, Spierdijk J and Breimer DD: Plasma concentrations of lidocaine and bupivacaine after subarachnoid administration. Anesthesiology 59: 191-195, 1983.
18. Denson DD, Bridenbaugh PO, Turner PA, Phero JC and Raj PP. Neural blockade and pharmacokinetics following subarachnoid lidocaine in the rhesus monkey. I. Effects of epinephrine. Anesth. Analg. 61: 746-750, 1982.

EFFECTS OF ADRENALINE DURING EPIDURAL AND SPINAL ANAESTHESIA

J.W. VAN KLEEF AND A.G.L. BURM

INTRODUCTION

Most of the actions of sympathomimetic agents can be classified into five types:
1. a peripheral excitatory action (alpha-effect)
   (on certain types of smooth muscles, e.g. bloodvessels
   supplying skin and mucous membranes)
2. a peripheral inhibitory action (beta$_2$-effect)
   (on other types of smooth muscles, e.g. bloodvessels in
   the wall of the gut; bronchial tree, and skeletal muscles)
3. a cardiac excitatory action (beta$_1$-effect)
   (increase of heart rate and force)
4. metabolic actions
   (increased glycogenolysis in the liver; liberation of
   FFA's)
5. CNS excitatory actions
   (respiratory stimulation; decreased appetite)
All sympathomimetic drugs do not show each of the above
mentioned actions to the same degree.
The prototype agent is adrenaline (epinephrine).
Adrenaline is produced in the adrenal medulla and acts upon
distant target organs. It has a wide variety of clinical uses
in medicine and surgery. In general these are based on the
actions of the drug on bloodvessels, heart and bronchial
musculature.
The most common indications for the use of adrenaline especially in anaesthesia are:
1. The relief of respiratory distress due to bronchospasm
2. To provide rapid relief of hypersensitivity reactions
3. To prolong the action of local anaesthetics.

EFFECTS ON HEART AND PERIPHERAL BLOODFLOW

If given rapidly intravenously adrenaline will evoke a
characteristic effect on blood pressure which will rise
rapidly to a peak proportional to the dose.[1] The increase in
systolic pressure will be greater than that of the diastolic
pressure. Thereafter the pressure will fall to below normal
before returning to the control level.[1] Minute doses of
adrenaline (0.1 μg/kg) may cause the blood pressure to fall.
This depressor effect of small doses and the biphasic
response to larger doses are due to a greater sensitivity of
vasodilator beta-receptors to adrenaline than that of vaso-

constrictor alpha-receptors. In addition larger doses acti-
vate alpha-receptors and the overall effect of full activa-
tion of both alpha- and beta-receptors is an increase in
peripheral resistance and consequently a rise in blood
pressure.

Adrenaline is not recommended as a vasopressor drug because
when rapidly administered intravenously in order to correct
the blood pressure it may produce anxiety, tachycardia and
cardiac irregularities even leading to ventricular fibrillation. On the other hand, Ephedrine (5-10 mg IV) or mephentermine (Wyamine[R], 15-30 mg IV) are vasopressors which are most
likely to be safe as well as practical under clinical conditions.[2] Their predominant beta-stimulating activity, increasing uterine perfusion pressure more than uterine vascular
resistance makes them the drug(s) of choice particularly in
obstetrics.[3]

As a result of the systemic absorption of small amounts of
adrenaline during epidural anaesthesia a marked increase in
cardiac output and a decrease in total peripheral resistance
may result. These changes in cardiovascular parameters can be
ascribed to a beta-receptor stimulating effect of adrenaline.
While the potential for cardiovascular changes owing to sympathetic block up to the same level is similar for epidural
and subarachnoid blockade, vascular absorption of local
anaesthetics and vasoconstrictors may result in significant
haemodynamic changes after epidural administration. Effects
of a high subarachnoid and a high epidural block with and
without adrenaline in the solution have been studied by Ward
et al.[4] In their study high subarachnoid block produced
hypotension, decreased stroke volume and cardiac output and
produced a slight decrease in peripheral resistance. High
epidural block with adrenaline in the anaesthetic solution
produced the same degree of hypotension but an increase in
heart rate, stroke volume and cardiac output and a marked
drop in peripheral resistance. High epidural block without
adrenaline in the local anaesthetic solution produced changes
similar to, but not as profound as, subarachnoid anaesthesia.
If during epidural anaesthesia a larger amount of adrenaline
reaches the systemic circulation such as after an inadvertent
intravascular injection of a 3 ml test dose of a local anaesthetic solution which contains 15 µg adrenaline, a
recognisable alpha- and beta-response of short duration will
be seen. Although a 3 ml dose of an appropriate concentration
of a local anaesthetic produces evidence of spinal anaesthesia within 2 minutes, definite evidence of an intravascular
injection will only become rapidly apparent if adrenaline is
added to the solution.[5] Of course the beta-effects will not
become clearly visible if the patient is on beta-blocker
therapy but the alpha-effects of adrenaline will become apparent in the form of a rise in blood pressure.

An unintentional inadvertent intravascular injection of a
full dose of a local anaesthetic during epidural anaesthesia
may lead to a systemic toxic reaction. Since the article by
Albright[6] in 1979 emphasis has been placed on the fact that
the longer acting local anaesthetic agents depress the myo-

cardium to a greater extent than the shorter acting local
anaesthetics. These myocardial depressant effects of local
anaesthetics during a systemic toxic reaction may be counter-
acted by the stimulatory effects of the added adrenaline on
the myocardium.[7]

INFLUENCE ON BLOOD FLOW AT THE SITE OF INJECTION

The rationale for combining adrenaline with a local
anaesthetic drug is to achieve vasoconstriction.
As a result of this:
1. the duration of action of certain local anaesthetic drugs
   may be prolonged by increased neuronal uptake of the local
   anaesthetic.
2. the rate of absorption of specific local anaesthetics from
   various sites of administration may be diminished.
During epidural anaesthesia the addition of adrenaline reduces the vascular absorption of the local anaesthetic to a
variable extent and enhances the efficacy of epidural
blockade. This is less marked, with the longer acting agents
bupivacaine and etidocaine. Adrenaline in a concentration of
1: 200.000 (= 5 µg/ml) may enhance the intensity of motor
blockade and the quality of sensory blockade at least in the
case of lidocaine and prilocaine.[8]
Also during spinal anaesthesia, vasoconstrictor agents may
prolong the duration of action of the local anaesthetic.
Meagher et al[9] found that adrenaline prolonged the action of
tetracaine during spinal anaesthesia but to a lesser extent
than phenylephrine. In a study by Moore[10] it was found that
adrenaline added to bupivacaine or tetracaine significantly
prolonged the duration of action of both drugs. In this study
the criterium for duration of sensory blockade was the onset
of pain in the operative side.
Chambers et al[11] found a statistical significant difference
with regard to total duration of the block but not with
regard to two and four segment regression produced by bupivacaine. In an earlier study Chambers et al[12] found similar
effects by adrenaline on spinal anaesthesia with lidocaine.
No differences were seen between the effects of adding 0,1;
0,2 or 0,3 ml of a 1:1000 adrenaline solution to a 5% lidocaine solution.

INVESTIGATIONS

In our study, we compared pharmacokinetic and clinical data
of plain versus adrenaline containing solutions of lidocaine
heavy (5% in 8% dextrose) and bupivacaine (0.5% in 8%
dextrose) after subarachnoid administration.

Methods

Each solution was administered to 10 patients. The patients
selected for inclusion in the study were those requiring
surgery of the lower extremity. As a 1:200.000 concentration
of adrenaline usually is employed, as an additive to local

anaesthetic solutions and assuming that adrenaline is diluted in about 30 ml of spinal fluid[13], 0.15 ml of a 1:1000 adrenaline solution was added to the local anaesthetic solution immediately before the block was performed. The nature of the solution used within the lidocaine and bupivacaine groups was only known to the anaesthetist performing the block. Each patient received 2 mg lorazepam sublingually one to two hours and 0.5 mg atropine intramuscularly 30 min before the procedure. Access to the subarachnoid space was obtained using a 25-gauge needle via the third lumbar interspace with the patient in the sitting position. Immediately after the solution was injected the patient was placed in a horizontal position. Analgesia was defined as the loss of sensation to pin-prick.

During our study we observed that the extension of the motor block followed a different pattern after spinal anaesthesia than what is commonly seen after epidural anaesthesia. Therefore we were unable to use the Bromage motor block classification. We classified the intensitiy of motor block by using a 3 point scale for each individual joint (hip, knee, ankle). No motor block was scored as zero; patial block was scored as one and total block was scored as two.

Central venous blood samples for the determination of the plasma levels were collected by means of a catheter introduced percutaneously via the cephalic vein. The location of the tip of the catheter was varified by means of a chest X-ray immediately before the block. The samples were collected before and at regular times after the injection. The plasma concentrations of the local anaesthetic were estimated with the aid of a gaschromatographic method described earlier by us.[14]

Results

There was no statistically significant difference in mean age, weight and height in the groups that were compared. Tables 1-4 show the clinical data; tables 5 and 6 show the pharmacokinetic data. The mean maximum cephalad spread of sensory loss (in time and segments) was not significantly different in the groups that were compared. The mean times taken until the block had regressed two and four segments were not significantly different comparing plain versus adrenaline containing solutions of lidocaine and bupivacaine.

Adrenaline had a significant effect ($p < 0.001$) on total duration of analgesia and total regression of motor block ($p < 0.05$) produced by lidocaine 5% as well as on the peak plasma concentration of lidocaine ($p < 0.02$).

Addition of adrenaline to bupivacaine 0,5% heavy did not result in a significant prolongation of the action and had no influence on the pharmacokinetic parameters.

TABLE 1 Data of sensory loss comparing plain versus adrenaline containing solutions of lidocaine 5%

	Lidocaine 5% hyperbaric (n=10)	Lidocaine 5% hyperbaric with adrenaline 0.15 ml 1:1000 (n=10)	Significance of difference
Initial onset (min)	<5	<5	N.S.
Max. spread (min)	20.5 + 15.2	16.1 + 7.0	N.S.
Max. spread (segment)	T 6.2 + 3.0	T 6.4 + 3.1	N.S.
2 segment regression* (min)	47.0 + 14.8	65.5 + 28.0	N.S.
4 segment regression* (min)	71.0 + 21.7	82.2 + 30.3	N.S.
Total regression* (min)	209 + 26	325 + 63	P<0.001

Values are means + S.D.

*Regression is expressed as the time of maximum cephalad spread of sensory loss to the time the level has regressed that respective number of segments.

TABLE 2   Data of sensory loss comparing plain versus adrenaline containing solutions of bupivacaine 0.5%

	Bupivacaine 0.5% hyperbaric (n=10)	Bupivacaine 0.5% hyperbaric with adrenaline 0.15 ml 1:1000 (n=10)	Significance of difference
Initial onset (min)	<5	<5	N.S.
Max. spread (min)	14.5 ± 3.7	15.6 ± 6.3	N.S.
Max. spread (segment)	T 7.3 ± 3.5	T 5.4 ± 2.4	N.S.
2 segment regression* (min)	66.3 ± 18.1	65.0 ± 29.4	N.S.
4 segment regression* (min)	98.9 ± 33.1	83.8 ± 38.6	N.S.
Total regression* (min)	386 ± 99	431 ± 110	N.S.

Values are means ± S.D.

*Regression is expressed as the time of maximum cephalad spread of sensory loss to the time the level has regressed that respective number of segments.

TABLE 3   Data of motor block comparing plain versus adrenaline containing solutions of lidocaine 5%

	Lidocaine 5% hyperbaric (n=10)	Lidocaine 5% hyperbaric with adrenaline 0.15 ml 1:1000 (n=10)	Significance of difference
Initial onset (min)	<6	<6	N.S.
Complete onset of block* (min)	9.0 ± 3.5	8.0 ± 4.8	N.S.
Complete block (% of patients)	90	70	N.S.
Total regression** (min)	113 ± 42	151 ± 24	$P < 0.05$

Values are means $\pm$ S.D.

*Complete onset of block is defined as the time from the injection to the time when the maximum degree of motor block was reached.

**Total regression is expressed as the time of complete onset of block to the time of complete recovery of the motor block.

TABLE 4   Data of motor block comparing plain versus adrenaline containing solutions of bupivacaine 0.5%

	Bupivacaine 0.5% hyperbaric (n=10)	Bupivacaine 0.5% hyperbaric with adrenaline 0.15 ml 1:1000 (n=10)	Significance of difference
Initial onset (min)	<6	<6	N.S.
Complete onset of block* (min)	13.5 ± 4.9	18.2 ± 9.1	N.S.
Complete block (% of patients)	70	80	N.S.
Total regression** (min)	156 ± 83	174 ± 79	N.S.

Values are means ± S.D.

*Complete onset of block is defined as the time from the injection to the time when the maximum degree of motor block was reached.

**Total regression is expressed as the time of complete onset of block to the time of complete recovery of the motor block.

TABLE 5   **Pharmacokinetic data comparing plain versus adrenaline containing solutions of lidocaine 5%**

	Lidocaine 5% hyperbaric (n=10)	Lidocaine 5% hyperbaric with adrenaline 0.15 ml 1:1000 (n=10)	Significance of difference
t_{max} (min)	71 ± 29	58 ± 24	N.S.
C_{max} (g/ml)	526 ± 141	362 ± 108	P<0.02
$t_{1/2}$el (h)	2.2 ± 0.6	2.7 ± 0.9	N.S.
AUC (mg.min/1)	115 ± 29	110 ± 33	N.S.
Cl (ml/min)	797 ± 220	841 ± 228	N.S.

TABLE 6   **Pharmacokinetic data comparing plain versus adrenaline containing solutions of bupivacaine 0.5%**

	Bupivacaine 0.5% hyperbaric (n=10)	Bupivacaine 0.5% hyperbaric with adrenaline 0.15 ml 1:1000 (n=10)	Significance of difference
t_{max} (min)	62 ± 33	59 ± 27	N.S.
C_{max} (g/ml)	70 ± 32	56 ± 15	N.S.
$t_{1/2}el$ (h)	4.7 ± 1.4	4.2 ± 1.1	N.S.
AUC (mg.min/1)	24.8 ± 12.0	23.5 ± 5.3	N.S.
Cl (ml/min)	606 ± 169	590 ± 130	N.S.

Discussion

In our investigation adrenaline had similar effects to that found by the Edinburgh group.[11,12]
The statistically significant difference in total regression of the bupivacaine block - with or without adrenaline - found by these investigators was not significant in our study. On the other hand, the addition of adrenaline to lidocaine lead in our investigation to a highly significant prolongation of the regression of the sensory blockade while the total regression of the motor block was merely significant. Our findings confirmed the general experience seen with the addition of adrenaline to local anaesthetics at other sites of injection, namely that the effect of adrenaline is greater when added to a short-acting local anaesthetic than when added to a long-acting agent.
The clinical effects we saw were also in accordance with the pharmacokinetic parameters measured by us in this investigation. In particular there was a significant lower Cmax observable after the addition of adrenaline to lidocaine. These lower plasma concentrations could perhaps be attributed to vasoconstriction at the site of injection. Theoretically it is also possible that systemic absorption of adrenaline and the resultant increase in cardiac output gives rise to an increased liver perfusion and thereby an increase in clearance of the local anaesthetic. The lower plasma concentrations which may result from this may be an additional factor, although this is improbable after subarachnoid administration. Consequently we have reached the conclusion that the observed adrenaline effects seen during subarachnoid block can be attributed to local vasoconstriction.
Another mechanism by which vasoconstrictors may prolong spinal anaesthesia may be by a direct pharmacologic action, rather than a physiologic one as has been shown by Kraynack et al.[15] They examined the local anaesthetic effects of adrenaline and ephedrine both in vivo and in vitro. 0,50 g of adrenaline produced reversible in vivo sciatic blocks in rats with a mean duration of 131 $\pm$ 10 min.
So the potentiation of local anaesthetic drugs in vivo may also be the result of a direct neural blocking action of adrenaline.

REFERENCES

1. Innes IR and Nickerson M. Norepinephrine, epinephrine and the sympathomimetic amines. In: The pharmacological basis of therapeutics, Eds. Goodman LS and Gilman A, 5th ed., 1975. MacMillan, New York/Toronto/London, pp. 477-514.
2. Greene NM. The cardiovascular system. In: physiology of spinal anesthesia, 3rd ed., 1981. Williams and Wilkins, Baltimore/London, pp. 63-147.
3. Snider SM. Vasopressors in obstetrics. Regional Anesthesia 8: 74-81, 1983.
4. Ward RJ, Bonica JJ, Freund FG, Akamatsu T, Danziger F and Englesson S. Epidural and subarachnoid anesthesia.

Cardiovascular and respiratory effects. JAMA 191: 275-279, 1965.
5. Moore DC, Batra MS. The components of an effective test dose prior to epidural block. Anesthesiology 55: 693-697, 1981.
6. Albright GA. Cardiac arrest following regional anesthesia with etidocaine or bupivacaine. Anesthesiology 51: 285-287, 1979.
7. Moore DC, Scurlock JE. Possible role of epinephrine in prevention or correction of myocardial depression associated with bupivacaine. Anesth. Analg. 62: 450-453, 1983.
8. Covino BG, Vassallo HG. Clinical aspects of local anesthesia. In: Local anesthetics mechanisms of action and clinical use. 1976. Grune and Stratton, New York/San Francisco/London, pp. 57-95.
9. Meagher RP, Moore DC, de Vries JC. Phenylephrine: the most potent potentiator of tetracaine spinal anesthesia. Anesth. Analg. 45: 134-139, 1966.
10. Moore DC. Spinal anesthesia: Bupivacaine compared with tetracaine. Anesth. Analg. 59: 743-750, 1980.
11. Chambers WA, Littlewood DG, Scott DB. Spinal anesthesia with hyperbaric bupivacaine: effect of added vasoconstrictors. Anesth. Analg. 61: 49-52, 1982.
12. Chambers WA, Littlewood DG, Logan MR, Scott DB. Effect of added epinephrine on spinal anesthesia with lidocaine. Anesth. Analg. 60:417-420, 1981.
13. Egbert LD, Deas TC. Effect of epinephrine upon the duration of spinal anesthesia. Anesthesiology 21: 345-347, 1960.
14. Burm AGL, van Kleef JW, de Boer AG. Gas chromatographic determination of bupivacaine in plasma using a support coated open tubular column and a nitrogen-selective detector. Anesthesiology 57:527-529, 1982.
15. Kraynack BJ, Gintautas J, Tjay H. Local anesthetic action of epinephrine and ephedrine. Regional Anesthesia 8: 32, 1983.

CARDIOVASCULAR EFFECTS OF EPIDURAL AND SPINAL BLOCK

D. B. SCOTT

Epidural and spinal block have similar but not identical effects on the cardiovascular system. Both affect the sympathetic outflow from the spinal cord to the sympathetic chain, and interfere with the sympathetic tone to the blood vessels and the heart. The sympathetic outflow derives from the spinal segments T1-L2 and the higher the block, the more sympathetic tone is affected. The heart is supplied from T1-5 and will only be affected by very high blocks. However it is also supplied with parasympathetic nerves from the vagi which will be unaffected by the blockade. Thus the heart will not only have its sympathetic tone reduced, but the parasympathetic nerves will be unopposed.

Because a much larger dose of local anaesthetic drug is used for epidural than spinal block there is, in the case of the former, the additional effect of the drug itself following absorption, together with that of any adrenaline that may have been added to it.

Thus we can divide the cardiovascular effects into those resulting from sympathetic blockade and those which are drug mediated.

Sympathetic blockade. Sympathetic tone varies widely from patient to patient. Much depends upon their state of anxiety and any co-incident disease state e.g. hypovolaemia.

Most normal individuals show little overall effects from a low block, although there will invariably be an increased blood flow to the lower limbs due to vasodilatation. This is compensated for by vasoconstriction in the upper limbs. The peripheral resistance being thus unaffected there is no fall in arterial pressure.

With higher blocks other vascular beds such as the renal and splanchnic become affected, the ability to vasoconstrict will be less and the arterial pressure will tend to fall. However most subjects can tolerate even very high blocks without a dangerous lowering of blood pressure,(1) provided their venous return is not obstructed, and their cardiac output is maintained. Blocks affecting the upper five thoracic segments will often cause a slowing of the heart. Should the heart rate be reduced to around 50 beats/min. then cardiac output will be reduced also and arterial pressure will fall.

Thus sympathetic blockade of itself may have three responses:-

a. Low blocks (below T10):- An increase in lower limb and a decrease in upper limb blood flow. No change in arterial pressure while supine or head down.

b. Medium blocks (T5-10):- Dilatation of splanchnic and renal arterial beds with decrease in total peripheral resistance. A moderate fall in arterial pressure but seldom requiring more than conservative treatment e.g. headdown posture and i.v. fluids.

c. High blocks (above T5):- Widespread vasodilation accompanied by bradycardia and a reduced cardiac output, with a fall in arterial pressure which may require treatment. Many patients will be relatively unaffected by high blocks, particularly if they are young. However some may require treatment. If the bradycardia and hypotension are not due to a vaso-vagal attack (vide infra) then they will respond to i.v. atropine (0.6 mg) or a vasoconstrictor e.g. ephedrine (15-30 mg).

Venous return. Veins are under the control of the sympathetic system and if this is blocked then venous tone is reduced and venous pressure will fall. It is often said that, as a result, pooling of blood will occur and venous return will decrease. Pooling however can only occur if the venous return is obstructed e.g. by the head-up posture or by inferior vena caval occlusion. If the patient is supine or head-down then venous return will be maintained. Any fall in arterial pressure will therefore be related to a decrease in peripheral resistance rather than cardiac output.

Vaso-vagal attack. Vaso-vagal fainting is a well known phenomenon, though it would appear to have no teleological purpose. It can be provoked by an upset in sympathetic/parasympathetic balance and is therefore not uncommon with epidural and spinal block. It is probably the most usual cause of the sudden and precipitous decrease in arterial pressure sometimes seen with these blocks. It is invariably accompanied by severe bradycardia (not infrequently with a short period of cardiac arrest). Consciousness may become clouded or lost. The patient may complain of nausea and vomiting may ensue. Often excessive sweating may occur.

Unlike the bradycardia due to high blocks, vaso-vagal attacks are resistant to atropine and it is better to treat them with vasoconstrictors.

They are not seen if the patient is receiving concomitant general anaesthesia.

Conditions pre-disposing to hypotension. Some patients are dependant upon a high sympathetic tone to maintain arterial pressure in the presence of a reduced cardiac output. A classical example is inferior vena caval pressure in late pregnancy. Most women can tolerate this provided they can vasoconstrict both arteries and veins to raise peripheral resistance and reduce venous capacitance. If sympathetic blockade prevents this compensation then arterial pressure will fall. About 25% of patients will become hypotensive during epidural blockade if kept supine during labour.

The same process can occur in other circumstances e.g. with other large abdominal tumours and in hypovolaemia due to loss of blood or body fluids. Thus patients with any degree of shock are extremely vulnerable to hypotension if epidural or spinal block is given.

Concomitant general anaesthesia. While this will prevent the sudden hypotension associated with vasovagal fainting, it is very frequently associated with a greater degree of hypotension than is seen in conscious patients (2). Most general anaesthetics are potent vasodilators and will further reduce peripheral resistance already lowered by the sympathetic nerve blockade. In addition some are capable of depressing the myocardium

especially if deep anaesthesia is used. However the hypotension is
of little danger to most patients and indeed it may be employed with
benefit to reduce operative bleeding.

The hypotension when it occurs is seldom if ever precipitate, usually
taking 20 - 30 minutes to become maximal.

Adrenaline.   The amount of adrenaline usually added to local anaesthetics
is seldom great (even with epidural blocks) and its effect after being
absorbed might be thought to be transient and feeble. However the changes
seen after plain solutions are given epidurally may be considerably
different to those seen after adding epinephrine to the local anaesthetic
solution (3). Heart rate and cardiac output are greater than with the
plain solution while arterial pressure is lower, especially in conscious
patients. The reasons for this are not clear but may well have something
to do with the fact that the initial absorption of the adrenaline resets
the levels of heart rate and arterial pressure which are maintained
long after the adrenaline is no longer active.

Local anaesthetic drugs. With epidural but not with spinal blocks, enough
local anaesthetic may be absorbed to affect the myocardium or the brain.
In low concentrations, agents such as lignocaine have a small but
definite positive inotropic effect, but as concentrations rise then
increasing myocardial depression becomes evident. This is seldom of
practical importance unless the drug has been given intravenously by
mistake when it is almost always preceded by signs of overt toxicity of
the central nervous system.

There is at present some dubiety regarding the potential of the drugs
bupivacaine and etidocaine for myocardial depression (4). This question
needs further elucidation, but a problem is only likely to arise if the
injection is given intravenously or an abnormally high dose is used.

Is hypotension dangerous? Induced hypotension is a technique which has
been used to reduce operative bleeding for nearly 40 years (5). Although
it has vigorous opponents, nevertheless it has been used in vast numbers
of patients without apparent harm. The two most feared complications are

cerebral hypoxia and coronary insufficiency. The former, if it occurs at all, must be extremely uncommon. However the myocardial blood supply is very dependent upon arterial pressure and reducing it is viewed with alarm especially if coronary artery disease is present, which of course it can be even in the absence of any signs or symptoms.

Induced hypotension should not be used in the conscious patient as it may well provoke a vasovagal attack and a period of extreme hypotension or even cardiac arrest may lead to a myocardial infarction in a patient with pre-existing disease.

If the patient is receiving a concomitant general anaesthetic and the arterial pressure is low with a normal or slightly reduced cardiac output, what are the constraints in regard to the coronary circulation? In a normal heart the reduced perfusion pressure is precisely matched with a reduction in cardiac work as each is linearly related to the mean arterial pressure, assuming the left ventricular end diastolic pressure is low. In the heart with coronary artery disease however, the position is much more complicated and it has to be admitted that at present we do not have the instruments to study regional myocardial blood supply adequately under induced hypotension. Monitoring the S-T segment of the electrocardiogram through the V5 lead will warn of increasing myocardial hypoxia but it may not be an early enough warning.

A further difficulty comes in deciding on how to correct the hypotension in this high risk group. Vasoconstrictors with both alpha and beta adrenergic stimulating properties such as ephedrine will greatly increase myocardial oxygen demand, perhaps more than the expected increase in oxygen supply. It may be that a drug such as methoxamine (which is an alpha stimulator but reduces cardiac output by slowing the heart rate) is a better choice, but this still awaits the proof of experiment.

Looked at from the opposite point of view, many anaesthetists are now much more wary of hypertension especially during intubation and surgery. Certainly the rate/pressure product is virtually never in the dangerous zone with spinal or epidural block especially if intubation (which is seldom required) is avoided.

Conclusion. The cardiovascular changes seen with epidural and spinal
anaesthesia require a proper understanding by the anaesthetist. He will
then be able either to use these changes to the patient's benefit or
correct them quickly and completely.

References

1. Bonica JJ, Berges PU, Morikawa K. Circulatory effects of peridural
    block: 1. Effects of level of analgesia and dose of lidocaine.
    Anesthesiology 1970;33:619-26.

2. Stephen GW, Lees MM, Scott DB. Cardiovascular effects of epidural
    block combined with general anaesthesia. Br J Anaesth 1969;41:993.

3. Stanton-Hicks M, Berges PU, Bonica JJ. Circulatory effects of
    peridural block: IV. Comparison of the effects of epinephrine and
    phenylephrine. Anesthesiology 1973;39:308-14.

4. Albright CA. Cardiac arrest following regional anaesthesia with
    etidocaine or bupivacaine (editorial views). Anesthesiol. 1979;51:285.

5. Griffiths HWC and Gilles J. Thoraco-lumbar splanchnicectomy and
    sympathectomy: Anaesthetic procedure. Anaesthesia 1948;3:134.

ABSORPTION AND DISPOSITION OF LOCAL ANAESTHETICS IN RELATION TO
REGIONAL BLOOD FLOW CHANGES

G.T. TUCKER

1. INTRODUCTION

Most of the clinically useful local anaesthetics are relatively
lipid-soluble compounds and, therefore, pass across biological membranes
without difficulty. Thus, delivery of the agents to such membranes
by the blood supply may rate-limit their pharmacokinetics. This is
particularly likely in the context of their systemic disposition once
absorption into the general circulation has taken place. However, both
diffusion and perfusion will play a role in translocation of local
anaesthetics at sites of injection.

This chapter will review the effects of changes in regional blood
flow as a determinant of the kinetics of local anaesthetics. Changes in
blood flow at sites of injection may have implications both for duration
of anaesthesia and systemic uptake and safety. Changes in peripheral
blood flow (other than at sites of injection) may influence the volume
of distribution of the drugs as a function of time, while variation in
the distribution of arm blood flow may alter arteriovenous concentration
differences of the agents with implications for the interpretation of
local anaesthetic 'blood levels'. Changes in hepatic blood flow could
have implications for the systemic elimination and , therefore, safety
of the agents.

Many factors may modify perfusion at these three sites. I shall
consider the effects of the local anaesthetic itself; of sympathetic
nerve block; of adrenaline; of disease, surgery and pregnancy and of
other anaesthetic and therapeutic agents. Although some experimental
data are available to support this discussion, much of our understanding
remains theoretical and speculative. Nevertheless, it is hoped that this
essay will stimulate further research in this area.

2. CARDIOVASCULAR EFFECTS OF LOCAL ANAESTHETICS

2.1. Direct action on vascular smooth muscle

At a local level it is well-established that local anaesthetics are vasoactive. Vasodilatation, for example, is readily demonstrated by an increase in limb blood flow following intra-arterial injection of the agents. On this basis bupivacaine and etidocaine are seen to produce more profound and prolonged effects than other anaesthetically less potent amides (1). Others have shown that these vasodilatory effects may, however, be converted to vasoconstriction in some vascular beds, particularly in the presence of a low tone of the vascular smooth muscle(2). Direct vasoconstrictor effects have also been shown with isolated vessel preparations, the order of potency being the opposite of that found in the limb blood flow studies - bupivacaine and etidocaine being the least vasoconstrictor (1). Either way, the evidence does then suggest that, of the available agents, bupivacaine and etidocaine are most likely to produce vasodilatation and mepivacaine and prilocaine are most likely to produce vasoconstriction.

Extrapolation of these findings to effects on blood flow at major sites of regional block is difficult, however. The relatively prolonged absorption of the long-acting local anaesthetics must be more a function of their local binding than of vascular activity since vasodilatation would tend to promote systemic uptake. Direct vascular regulation of absorption may be a more important factor for the short-acting agents such as lignocaine and prilocaine.

2.2. Systemic cardiovascular effects

Changes in regional blood flow caused by systemically mediated effects of local anaesthetics may also influence their own absorption and disposition. Thus, below a threshold associated with convulsions and myocardial depression, which would decrease perfusion, the systemic presence of local anaesthetics causes an increase in cardiac output and blood pressure (3-5). The mechanism of this effect is probably a combination of an evoked increase in sympathetic activity in the C.N.S. and the direct venoconstrictor action in certain vascular beds already mentioned. The implication of this effect is that, if these changes are reflected in local perfusion pressures, this might enhance the absorption of local anaesthetic. On the other hand, distribution and elimination may also be speeded, the latter change being mediated by an increase in hepatic perfusion. Thus, Wiklund (3,4) has shown that short-term i.v. infusions of 2mg/min bupivacaine and etidocaine and 4mg/min lignocaine are all associated with a progressive rise (to about 25-30% of control) in hepatic blood flow.

3.   CARDIOVASCULAR EFFECTS OF SYMPATHETIC NERVE BLOCK
     Superimposed on the cardiovascular effects of local anaesthetics per se will be the cardiovascular effects of the nerve block that they produce.

     For example, following the injection of plain solutions (e.g. 400mg lignocaine) for T5 epidural anaesthesia, systemic cardiovascular effects are relatively minor in conscious volunteer subjects. There is a small fall in arterial blood pressure due primarily to a decrease in peripheral vascular resistance, with little change in cardiac output and a slight rise in heart rate (6). This presumably reflects the balance of the opposing effects of the cardiostimulatory influence of circulating drug and the effects of the sympathetic block. With higher doses of local anaesthetic the greater blood drug concentrations may result in a significant increase in cardiac output. With higher blocks a greater degree of hypotension will be obtained. The net effects on perfusion of the epidural space, systemic uptake of local anaesthetic and duration of anaesthesia are difficult to predict.

     Light general anaesthesia in fit patients does not materially affect the cardiovascular response to lumbar epidural anaesthesia (T5?) with plain local anaesthetic solutions (7).

     Despite the rather unremarkable effects of a T5 block on blood pressure and cardiac output, hepatic blood flow may be decreased by as much as 30% (8). Apparently, therefore, this effect is independent of cardiac output. There must be an additional influence of sympathetic block directly on the liver and this effectively overrides any stimulant effects of the circulating local anaesthetic. The implication here is that, to the extent that it is dependent upon hepatic perfusion, the systemic clearance of local anaesthetic may be delayed. Unfortunately, there are no data to substantiate this, at least for T5 block. There are data, however, showing that a T6-T7 block with tetracaine does not influence the systemic disposition kinetics of intravenous etidocaine (9). In monkeys Sivarajan et al (10) observed significant falls in coronary, hepatic, renal and cerebral blood flows during T1 epidural anaesthesia. These changes would certainly be expected to have a profound influence on local anaesthetic kinetics.

Apart from effects on central haemodynamics, epidural block also causes changes in peripheral blood flows. Thus, lumbar sympathetic block results in vasodilatation in the legs with compensatory vasoconstriction in the arms and a lowering of arm blood flow (6). This is reflected in considerable arteriovenous concentration differences in plasma concentrations of local anaesthetics - that across the arm being much greater than that

across the leg (9). It becomes important then to measure arterial concentrations of local anaesthetics in pharmacokinetic studies of regional anaesthesia since these should give a better indication of the time-profiles of the agents in well-perfused vital organs.

4. CARDIOVASCULAR EFFECTS OF ADRENALINE

The local effects of adrenaline on the systemic uptake of local anaesthetics are well-documented (11). Not only do the effects vary considerably with the site of injection and its vascularity but they also depend upon the particular local anaesthetic. For example, after epidural injection adrenaline markedly lowers peak plasma concentrations of mepivacaine and lignocaine but has little effect on those of prilocaine and etidocaine. The lack of effect on prilocaine may be due to the inherent vasoconstrictor properties of this agent while the lack of effect on etidocaine may reflect an overriding importance of tissue binding on the absorption of this compound. The fact that mepivacaine has the greatest intrinsic vasoconstrictor potency of the amides is difficult to reconcile with an influence of adrenaline on its absorption.

In addition to its local effect, adrenaline also has systemic effects which significantly modify the cardiovascular response to epidural anaesthesia. For example, an increase in cardiac output of 30-50%, a 40% decrease in peripheral resistance and a 20% decrease in mean arterial pressure were observed in conscious volunteers during T5 block achieved with 400mg lignocaine plus 1:200,000 adrenaline (6). The marked increase in cardiac output and decrease in peripheral resistance were assigned to the beta$_1$- and beta$_2$-adrenoceptor stimulant effects of absorbed adrenaline, although the prolonged time-course of these changes led Scott et al (12) to suggest that they may reflect a resetting of autonomic balance rather than any persistence in the circulation of the adrenaline. Whatever the mechanism, it is conceivable that these systemic cardiovascular effects of adrenaline could interact with its local vasoconstrictor action in modulating the uptake of local anaesthetics from sites of injection. Changes in the systemic clearance of local anaesthetics might also be anticipated since the beta-effects of adrenaline result in an increased liver blood flow (mediated partly through its direct influence on cardiac output and, perhaps, by direct interaction with intra-hepatic beta$_2$- receptors). Studies in both monkeys (13) and in man (8) showed that adrenaline absorbed from the epidural space at least temporarily offsets the lowering of hepatic blood flow caused by sympathetic blockade.

5. CARDIOVASCULAR EFFECTS OF DISEASE/SURGERY/PREGNANCY

Clearly the cardiovascular effects of regional anaesthesia and the implications for local anaesthetic kinetics are complex, being a function of the extent of sympathetic block, the systemic plasma concentration of local anaesthetic and the presence or absence of adrenaline in the injected solution. Most of the studies mentioned so far have involved normal volunteers. The pathophysiological status of the patient must also be considered.

5.1. Blood loss

There is evidence to suggest a relationship between the extent of surgical blood loss and the duration of regional anaesthesia (14). The most likely explanation for this is impaired perfusion at the site of injection and slowed systemic absorption of the local anaesthetic. Thus, a study in dogs showed a marked lowering of peak plasma lignocaine concentrations after epidural injection following acute hypovolaemia (15). Haemorrhage has also been shown to impair the systemic clearance of lignocaine in monkeys during i.v. infusion (16).

5.2. Heart failure and liver disease

Both of these conditions have been shown to be associated with a 50% decrease in the clearance of lignocaine together with changes in its volume of distribution (decreased in heart failure; increased in liver disease (17). In part, these changes are mediated by alteration in hepatic blood flow and in the distribution of the cardiac output. It might be expected that heart failure would slow the systemic absorption of local anaesthetics after regional block, but this has not been investigated.

5.3. Renal disease

In keeping with the liver being the major organ of elimination for local anaesthetics, the disposition kinetics of lignocaine were found to be minimally affected by renal disease (17). If anything, systemic clearance was slightly increased, possibly reflecting the hyperdynamic circulation in many of these patients and an increase in liver blood flow. Bromage and Gertel (18) have suggested that increased peripheral blood flow in patients with renal failure might account for a markedly shorter duration of brachial plexus block - due to faster systemic absorption of local anaesthetic.

5.4. Pregnancy

It is well-known that epidural dosage requirements are lowered in pregnant women and, in part, this might be explained by an increased systemic drug absorption rate resulting from a hyperdynamic circulation and engorgement of the epidural veins. However, no significant differences were observed in plasma drug concentration - time profiles after epidural injection of etidocaine in pregnant women at term and in a group of older, non-pregnant patients (19). Nevertheless, increases in absorption and elimination may cancel each other out during pregnancy.

6. CARDIOVASCULAR EFFECTS OF OTHER DRUGS

By altering local, peripheral or hepatic blood flows other drugs can also influence the kinetics of local anaesthetics.

6.1. Changes in local blood flow

It has been proposed that i.v. injection of ephedrine, by increasing cardiac output and arterial blood pressure, might increase the rate of systemic absorption of local anaesthetic (20).

6.2. Changes in peripheral blood flow

Arteriovenous concentration differences of local anaesthetics across the arm after epidural injection of the agents were found to be less in patients than in volunteer subjects (9). This raised the possibility that premedication of the former, by causing a generalised vasodilatation, might have antagonised compensatory vasoconstriction in the arm following blockade. Preliminary data (Mather et al - in preparation) lend some substance to this hypothesis. Thus, arteriovenous concentration differences in plasma lignocaine were generally smaller in volunteer subjects when epidural injection of the local anaesthetic was preceeded by an i.m. injection of 100mg pethidine than when it was not.

6.3. Changes in hepatic blood flow

Mean values for the systemic blood clearance of the amide-type local anaesthetics in normal subjects increase in the order: bupivacaine (0.58 L/min), mepivacaine (0.78 L/min), lignocaine (0.95 L/min), etidocaine (1.11 L/min), prilocaine (2.37 L/min) (11). With the exception of the value for the latter which exceeds liver blood flow (1.5 L/min), suggesting some extrahepatic metabolism, these values essentially represent hepatic drug clearance (21). Accordingly, etidocaine is seen to have a high hepatic extraction ratio (0.74), those of lignocaine and mepivacaine are intermediate (0.5-0.6) and that of bupivacaine (0.4) is relatively low. Therefore, according to well-established pharmacokinetic principles (22), changes in hepatic blood flow are most likely to influence the disposition kinetics of etidocaine, those of lignocaine and mepivacaine are partially flow-dependent whereas the kinetics of bupivacaine should be sensitive predominantly to changes in the activity of drug metabolising enzymes. This classification should be borne in mind when interpreting mechanisms of pharmacokinetically-based drug interactions with local anaesthetics.

A number of drugs are known to modify the systemic clearance of lignocaine at least partly through their effects on hepatic perfusion.

6.3.1. Sympathomimetics

The effects of adrenaline have already been considered. Benowitz et al (16) have documented the influence of noradrenaline (alpha-adrenoceptor stimulation) and of isoprenaline (beta-adrenoceptor stimulation) on the disposition kinetics of lignocaine in monkeys. The former significantly increased half-life, decreased initial volume of distribution and decreased clearance by lowering hepatic blood flow; the latter produced exactly opposite effects.

In man, Wiklund et al (23) have shown that an i.v. injection of 20mg ephedrine significantly increased hepatic blood flow and , thereby, the clearance of intravenous lignocaine. Whether this also happens in the presence of sympathetic blockade is not known.

6.3.2. Halothane

In dogs, hepatic clearance of lignocaine was significantly lowered under halothane anaesthesia compared to nitrous oxide (24). Decreases in both hepatic blood flow and in mixed function oxidase activity are probably responsible for the inhibitory effect of halothane.

6.3.3. Cimetidine

This drug has been shown to decrease the volume of distribution of lignocaine in man and to lower its clearance by up to 25-40% (25,26). Again, the mechanism is believed to be a combination of effects on hepatic perfusion and enzyme activity. In contrast, ranitidine, an alternative H_2-receptor antagonist, does not appear to influence lignocaine kinetics (27).

6.3.4. Beta-adrenoceptor antagonists

Propranolol has been shown to lower the clearance of lignocaine in man (28-30). The mechanism of this effect was originally attributed solely to a decrease in hepatic blood flow secondary to lowering of cardiac output by the beta-blocker. However, the extent of the change is greater than the anticipated reduction in hepatic perfusion and in vitro studies using both rat and human liver microsomes have shown an additional effect due to direct inhibition of the oxidation of lignocaine (31,32).

Studies in normal volunteers with other beta-blockers indicate that metoprolol also lowers lignocaine clearance but to a lesser extent than propranolol (30), while the effect of pindolol is minimal (29). The latter finding was attributed to the partial agonist activity of pindolol which causes a small rise rather than a fall in cardiac output in resting subjects. The in vitro studies with liver microsomes (31,32) show a strong correlation between the lipid-solubility of beta-blockers and their ability to inhibit the metabolism of lignocaine. Theoretical pharmaco-kinetic calculations based upon likely changes in hepatic blood flow and intrinsic clearance of lignocaine produced by the various beta-blockers predict observed changes in total lignocaine clearance with reasonable accuracy (32).

These effects of beta-blockers on the disposition kinetics of
lignocaine have obvious implications for the i.v. dosage of the latter
for the treatment and prevention of ventricular dysrhythmias since the
combination of these drugs is increasingly common. How the haemodynamic
response to regional anaesthesia and the pharmacokinetics of local
anaesthetics might be modified in patients receiving therapy with beta-
blockers and other drugs with potent cardiovascular activity remains to
be investigated.

7. CONCLUSIONS

The effects of changes in regional blood flow accompanying anaesthesia
on the absorption and disposition kinetics of local anaesthetics, as well
as those of other drugs given in the perioperative period, involve a
large number of variables. Currently, our understanding in this area is
limited and further advances will require carefully designed experiments.
This probably means going to an animal model where all of the variables
can be tightly controlled. A start in this direction has been made using
sheep and preliminary data comparing the haemodynamic and pharmacokinetic
effects of spinal ($\geq$ T4 with fluid preload) and general anaesthesia
(thiopentone/halothane1.5%) have been published (33). In these studies,
only general anaesthesia was shown to be associated with marked decreases
in the hepatic, renal and pulmonary clearance of model drugs (pethidine,
cefoxitin, chlormethiazole). Further systematic investigation of this
kind using epidural as well as spinal anaesthesia is clearly indicated.

REFERENCES

1.   Blair MR. 1975. Cardiovascular pharmacology of local anaesthetics.
     Br.J.Anaesth., 47 (Suppl.): 247-252.
2.   Aberg G, Dhuner KG. 1972. Effects of mepivacaine (Carbocaine) on
     femoral blood flow in the dog. Acta Pharmacol. Toxicol.)Kbh.), 31:
     267-271.
3.   Wiklund L. 1977a. Human hepatic blood flow and its relation to
     systemic circulation during intravenous infusion of lidocaine.
     Acta Anaesth.Scand., 21: 148-160.
4.   Wiklund L. 1977b. Human hepatic blood flow and its relation to
     systemic circulation during intravenous infusion of bupivacaine or
     etidocaine. Acta Anaesth. Scand., 21: 189-199.
5.   Martin MA, Bax NDS, Tucker GT, Ward JW. 1980. Disopyramide and
     lignocaine: A comparison of cardiac effects using echocardiography.
     Br.J.Clin.Pharmacol., 10: 237-244.
6.   Stanton-Hicks M d'A. 1975. Cardiovascular effects of extradural

7. Germann PAS, Roberts JG, Prys-Roberts C. 1979. The combination of general anaesthesia and epidural block 1: The effects of sequence of induction on haemodynamic variables and blood gas measurements in healthy patients. Anaesth. Int. Care, 7: 229-238.
8. Kennedy WF, Everett GB, Cobb LA, Allen GD. 1971. Simultaneous systemic and hepatic hemodynamic measurements during high peridural anesthesia in normal men. Anesth. Analg.:Curr.Res., 50: 1069-1077.
9. Tucker GT, Mather LE. 1975. Pharmacokinetics of local anaesthetic agents. Br.J.Anaesth., 47 (Suppl.): 213-224.
10. Sivarajan M, Amory DW, Lindbloom LE. 1976. Systemic and regional blood flow during epidural anesthesia without epinephrine in the rhesus monkey. Anesthesiology 45: 300-310.
11. Tucker GT, Mather LE. 1979. Clinical pharmacokinetics of local anaesthetics. Clin. Pharmacokin., 4: 241-278.
12. Scott DB, Littlewood DG, Drummond GB, Buckley PF, Covino BG. 1977. Modification of the circulatory effects of extradural block combined with general anaesthesia by the addition of adrenaline to lignocaine solutions. Br.J.Anaesth., 49: 917-925.
13. Amory DW, Sivarajan M, Lindbloom LE. 1977. Systemic and regional blood flow during epidural anesthesia with epinephrine in the rhesus monkey. Acta Anaesth. Scand., 21: 423-429.
14. Quimby CW. 1965. Influence of blood loss on the duration of regional anesthesia. Anesth. Analg.:Curr. Res., 44: 387-390.
15. Morikawa KI, Bonica JJ, Tucker GT, Murphy TM. 1974. Effects of acute hypovolaemia on lignocaine absorption and cardiovascular response following epidural block in dogs. Br.J.Anaesth., 46: 631-635.
16. Benowitz NL, Forsyth RP, Melmon KL, Rowland M. 1974. Lidocaine disposition kinetics in monkey and man. II. Effects of hemorrhage and sympathomimetic drug administration. Clin.Pharmacol.Ther., 16: 99-109.
17. Thomson PD, Melmon KL, Richardson JA, Cohn K, Steinbrunn W, Cudihee R, Rowland M. 1973. Lidocaine pharmacokinetics in advanced heart failure, liver disease and renal failure in humans. Ann.Int.Med., 78: 499-508.
18. Bromage PR, Gertel M. 1972. Brachial plexus anesthesia in chronic renal failure. Anesthesiology 36: 488-493.
19. Morgan DH, Cousins MJ, McQuillan D, Thomas J. 1977. Disposition and placental transfer of etidocaine in pregnancy. Eur.J.Clin.Pharmacol., 12: 359-365.
20. Mather LE, Tucker GT, Murphy TM, Stanton-Hicks M, Bonica JJ. 1976. Haemodynamic drug interaction: peridural lignocaine and intravenous ephedrine. Acta Anaesth. Scand., 20: 207-210.
21. Tucker GT, Wiklund L, Berlin-Wahlen A, Mather LE. 1977. Hepatic clearance of local anaesthetics in man. J.Pharmacokin. Biopharm., 5: 111-122.
22. Tucker GT. 1981. Principles of Pharmacokinetics. In: Therapeutic Drug Monitoring (eds. A Richens, V.Marks), London and Edinburgh, Churchill-Livingstone, pp 31-53.
23. Wiklund L, Tucker GT, Engberg G. 1977. Influence of intravenously administered ephedrine on splanchnic haemodynamics and clearance of lidocaine. Acta Anaesth. Scand., 21: 275-281.
24. Burney RG, Di Fazio CA. 1976. Hepatic clearance of lidocaine during N_2O anesthesia in dogs. Anesth. Analg.:Curr.Res., 55: 322-325.
25. Féely J, Wilkinson GR, McAllister CB, Wood AJJ. 1982. Increased

toxicity and reduced clearance of lidocaine by cimetidine. Ann.Int. Med., 96: 592-593.

26. DiFazio CA, Moscicki JC, DiFazio CJ. 1982. Cimetidine inhibits lidocaine plasma clearance. Anesthesiology 57: A188.

27. Feely J, Guy E. 1983. Lack of effect of ranitidine on the disposition of lignocaine. Br.J.Clin.Pharmacol., 15: 378-379.

28. Ochs HR, Carstens G, Greenblatt DJ. 1980. Reduction in lidocaine clearance during continuous infusion and by coadministration of propranolol. New Eng.J.Med., 303: 373-377.

29. Svendsen TL, Tango M, Waldorff S, Steiness E, Trap-Jensen J. 1982. Effects of propranolol and pindolol on plasma lignocaine clearance. Br.J.Clin.Pharmacol., 13: 223S-226S.

30. Conrad KA, Byers JM, Finley PR, Burnham L. 1983. Lidocaine elimination: Effects of metoprolol and of propranolol. Clin.Pharmacol.Ther.,33: 133-138.

31. Deacon CS, Lennard MS, Bax NDS, Woods HF, Tucker GT. 1981. Inhibition of oxidative drug metabolism by beta-adrenoceptor antagonists is related to their lipid-solubility. Br.J.Clin.Pharmacol., 12: 429-431.

32. Tucker GT, Bax NDS, Lennard MS, Al-Asady S, Bharaj HS, Woods HF. 1983. Effects of beta-adrenoceptor antagonists on the pharmacokinetics of lignocaine. Br.J.Clin.Pharmacol., in press.

33. Mather LE, Runciman WB, Ilsley AH. 1982. Anesthesia-induced changes in regional blood flow: implications for drug disposition. Regional Anesthesia 7(Suppl.): S24-S37.

MECHANISMS OF PAIN

JOH. SPIERDIJK

INTRODUCTION

In spite of the fact that much is written about mechanisms of pain, there is in my opinion no mechanism of pain.

Theories about pain are changing every twenty years and since the Mellzack and Wall Theory of pain mechanisms exist 18 years - we expect a new theory in the next few years, perhaps with the title "no mechanisms of pain".

In the Bonica lecture of 1979 Wall describes three stages of pain, the immediate, the acute and the chronic pain, linked less to injury than to body state. According to Wall pain is more an awareness of a need situation (like hunger) than an awareness of an event situation (like seeing). Pain itself can be linked casually to injury, it need not be, injury does not always generate pain, nor does pain always signal injury. Wall points out that seeing and hearing, sensations related to external events, enable us to describe quite accurately the location, duration, and strength of the external stimulus; whereas hunger and thirst, sensory experiences evoked by internal events, not only are difficult to describe precisely, but also are affected strongly by one's emotional state. The same is true with pain: often the stimulus is unknown, and the source mis-localized. Pain, though it profoundly affects us, seldom tells us its cause. Assuming all along the pain serves some sort of informative function, what then is its role? In the Leiden Pain Control Unit we learned that the relationship between cause and pain was unpredictable. For the patient, other factors besides the disease are involved! These factors are mainly affective and emotional in nature, for instance:

FEAR:
Fear of the diagnosis, fear about the effectiveness of the therapy, fear of the future (both his own and that of his family), and fear of the pain still to come.

EXPERIENCE:
Experience with pain, the same pain that made an operation or irradiation necessary.

REACTIONS OF THOSE AROUND THE PATIENT:
How do they react, what do they want to know about what the patient is experiencing, are they afraid of developing the same disease, do they show exaggerated concern or cheerfulness?

PERSONALITY:
The patient's personality of course plays an important part

in how he experiences the pain.

All these points must be taken into account when pain control is attempted in these patients. They need a doctor who does not only give an analgesic but also attention and guidance. Guidance of the patient must be provided by the physician in collaboration with relatives, friends or services set up especially for this purpose.

Wall in his lecture pointed out the following stages of pain:
1. The immediate pain as a direct response to injury followed by
2. Acute pain. During this acute phase of pain the patient is coping with the cause of injury and prepares himself for recovery. It is dominated by pain and by anxiety for the past, the present and the future. Acute anxiety is as much a point of this phase as is acute pain.

The third or chronic phase of pain is marked by recovery from injury, quiet inactivity being Nature's way of providing optimal conditions for healing. The great majority of injured people recover. But in a few patients without permanent injury the chronic phase drags on far beyond the necessity of recovery. It is this extreme of a natural sequence of events that provides the setting for the chronic pain syndrome.

Intractable pain, together with depression and lassitude, characterizes the extreme of the chronic phase. Behaviour changes, the patient focusing more and more on his condition and less and less on his surroundings. Complaints seem to be unremitting, depression deepens, and the search for treatment begins to dominate life. As the original signs of injury or disease have resolved long since, here again is a mismatch between amount of pain and amount of injury. And, as we cannot find anything wrong organically to match up with the very apparent distress of the patient, chronic pain is all too often relegated to the "it's all in your mind" category.

The same holds for the scientific investigation of the "intractable pain" syndrome. "By definition, an intractable pain patient cannot be treated", at least if we start from the fiction that the doctor or the team know everything about pain. But we actually know little more about pain than that, as Sternbach but it, "Pain is a hurt that we feel".

Intractable pain is not always intractable. It is only intractable when no success can be obtained with an integrated approach, as opposed to failure with a single approach. And even in these cases of failure the patient can be given substantial help, support, and guidance in his struggle with the pain. Conversely, an intractable patient can only be considered cured if the effect of the treatment lasts longer than a specified time, and this brings me to another difficult point. In the treatment of intractable pain patients and for the discussion and comparison of the results, it is necessary to agree on a follow-up period of, in my opinion, at least a year. Only then one can say whether the treatment is really effective and whether there is hope of a "cure". Our treatment can fail not only in a patient with an incurable disease but also in patients with a diagnosis for which, in our view, the pain experienced is out of proportion to the somatic anomalies or - which is even more difficult for us as physicians - in cases in which we can find no cause at all for the pain. Sometimes we achieve a temporary success. This transient success is dependent on many factors. In our opinion, one of these factors is the promotion of a given form of treatment. We believe that the temporary success of a certain treatment applied to the body can make the patient receptive to a more specific form of psychotherapy. We must never lose sight of the fact that pain is often an expression of a disintegration of the patient in relation to his or her partner and/or his or her world.

If you decide to work in a nerve block clinic you can certainly do worthwhile work there. If at the same time you are interested in psycho-social problems, and have a lot of time, any one of you can accomplish a great deal in the alleviation of pain and the guidance of pain patients. The combined knowledge of a pain group is much greater, even though it is still inadequate; but we continue to learn every day. Although none of us has sufficient knowledge or time.

The crux of the problem is indicated by the American expression T.L.C., or tender loving care, words which underline once again what many pain patients need. Perhaps the future will bring it. But instead of T.L.C., many physicians prefer the knife or the needle. In addition, they feel unable to trust the judgement of the doctors who have already seen the patient.

What the patient needs primarily is time and attention. This confronts us with the question of whether every patient who comes to us must be treated.
The following case is a good example of "it's pain when it hurts". Patient A is a man with brachialgia. He says that he wants to work but cannot. The doctor says he can carry 80% of his former load. So he works, but don't ask how. He has seen many doctors but they have not been able to do much for him. Our rheumatologist commented: "In our opinion, much too much diagnosis and therapy have been committed on this man". We gave him transcutaneous nerve stimulation; he said the effect was incredible. But then, after the third talk with him, we learned that even though he no longer had any pain he still only had to work 80% of full time: there was too little work for too many people. With transcutaneous nerve stimulation and psychotherapy we can give him further help. This patient is a man who reacted with pain to a phenomenon which Laurence Peter and Raymond Hull describe as the "Final Placement Syndrome" in their book The Peter Principle. Peter and Hull analysed hierachiology, and they think that "every organization contains a number of persons who could not do their jobs. These employees have been promoted from a position in which they were competent to a position in which they are incompetent". The authors' conclusion that every employee tends to rise to his level of incompetence, forms what is now

widely known as the Peter principle.

The level of incompetence does not always have to be a very
high one. The principle holds equally well for lower level
occupations and is just as valid for households and the
family. It certainly holds for husbands and wives. Peter
comes to the conclusion that placement at the level of incompetence can lead to pathology.
The following quotation from the book called <u>The Peter Prin-
ciple</u> is highly relevant in this context:
to recognize the existence of the Final Placement Syndrome!
In fact, that profession has displayed a frigid hostility
towards my application of hierachiology to the pseudo-science
of diagnostics. However, truth will out! Time and the increasingly tumultuous social order inevitably will bring
enlightenment.
Peter argues that two medical errors are made:
Futile approach.
Final Placement Syndrome patients often rationalize the situation: they claim their occupational incompentence is the
result of their physical ailments. "If only I could get rid
of these headaches, I could concentrate on my work".
Or "If only I could get my digestion fixed up..." and so on.
Some medical men accept this rationalization at face
value, and attack the physical symptoms without any search
for their cause.
This attack is made by medication or surgery, either of
which may give temporary, <u>but only temporary</u>, relief. The
patient cannot be drugged into competence and there is no
tumour of incompetence which can be removed by a stroke of
the scalpel. <u>Good advice</u> is equally ineffective.
"Take it easy"
"Don't work so hard"
"Learn to relax"
Such soothing suggestions are useless. Many F.P.S. patients
feel anxious because they now quite well that they are doing
very little useful work. They are unlikely to follow any
suggestion that they should do still less.
The second medical error lies in the non-existence
approach. A second group of physicians, finding nothing organically wrong with an F.P.S. patient, will try to persuade
him that <u>his symptoms do not exist!</u>
"There is really nothing wrong with you. Just take these
tranquillizers."
"Get your mind off yourself. These symptoms are only
imaginary. It's your nerves."
Such advice, of course, produces no lasting improvement.
The patient <u>knows that he is suffering</u>, whether the physician
will admit it or not.

We have all seen these patients in our practice: out of
place in their jobs, out of place in their families, out of
place in their surroundings. Other work, less work, reorgani-
zation of work, early retirement...everything has been
considered? The behaviour therapists will have to tell us

what the right treatment is.

It is sometimes difficult for non-psychiatrists and non-psychologists to accept that the diagnosis may also be psychiatric and it sometimes creates difficulties for the patient as well.

The following case history is an example:
A married woman with five children, and a husband in a high position, complained of pain in her tongue. She was sent from doctor to doctor and she was given all possible drugs. Injections with local anaesthetics, and even with alcohol, into her tongue, did not relieve the pain; on the contrary, the pain in her tongue still remained.

After cryosurgery of the nervus lingualis, a partial tongue resection was performed, and still there was no relief from pain. This patient was not helped with drugs, knives or needles.

The psychiatrist in our Paingroup was asked to treat this woman; he reduced the enormous number of drugs she was taking, and he started his own therapy. Now she is much better. There is less pain and she is back at home, leading a normal life.

Another patient was a good-looking sportsman. He had low-back pain and wanted to be treated like his colleague and be operated upon. But his family doctor refused to send him to the neurosurgeon. With Christmas he addressed himself to the pain clinic, totally helpless and confused. After a multidisciplinary approach to this man, it turned out that he was in financial trouble and an alcoholic and that he had family problems and also some pain.

With rest, fysiotherapy and the help of the psychiatrist and of the social worker, we could help this patient without an operation.

But don't forget, the opposite is also possible.

Patient 4 was a well-known professor. He became director of a very big plant, but it tunred out that he was not a manager of industry. He returned to the university and began to complain about pain in his neck.

The doctors started thinking that the pain in his neck had a mental origin (The Peter Principle). He had consultations in a small town-hospital, but no diagnosis was made. He went to the paramedical profession and they cracked his neck. Later on the doctor prescribed him a liss of Glisson for a few hours a day.

When this man entered my office, I realized immediately that he was very ill. He was extremely anxious and could hardly move his neck. We took him to our clinic and started investigations. Our neurologist was not sure about the diagnosis and ordered X-rays. During the night the patient developed a quadriplegia. X-rays showed destruction of the corpus of cervical 4 and a total blockage at that level by myelography; C3-C4-C5 had been partly destroyed by a malignant process. The patient was operated upon and a bone transplant of the os ilium was used to stabilize the neck. Pathological investigation revealed metastases from a bronchogenic carcinoma.

The patient died a few days after the operation.

SUMMARY

The mechanisms of pain are very complicated and the pain patient is difficult to treat. Before starting any kind of therapy it is wise to look into the emotional factors, such as their relationships with their partners, and their working circumstances.

Carron states that the health system in the USA offers the chronic pain patient "a sequential, specialty evaluation and treatment modality, indigenous to the specialty itself. This private consultation referral system frequently ends in further drug habituation or exploring surgery. Seldom are the emotional, social, family and occupational problems confronting the patient into account under such a system."

I think this is true for all Western countries.

CONCLUSION

Our conclusion can be seen in the light of what Sternbach wrote as early as 1966: "Any technique that dissociates the stimuli and responses, whether physical, chemical, behavioral or subjective, or whatever, can serve to alleviate pain. We need not be bound by traditions but are limited only by our imaginations."

We are of the opinion that an anaesthetist can play an important part in pain control. He will do so mainly in the field of nerve blocks. An anaesthetist who wants to do more than this, will have to make a study of the pain syndromes and the psyche of the patient. In addition, he can make an important contribution as a member of a multidisciplinary team.

General rules concerning the attitude towards patients who suffer from chronic pain are difficult to give in these circumstances, because each patient need his own therapy. But there are a few factors that you must never forget and I will give them as recommendations.

RECOMMENDATIONS

The basic principles for handling the mechanisms of pain treatment are:
1. Try to find a diagnosis.
2. Try to form a multidisciplinary pain group.
3. Give enough time to the patient and to the pain group.
4. Take enough time to study pain syndromes.
5. Try to find a curative method to take the pain away.
6. Do not play with the patient's psyche if you are not trained as a psychiologist or a psychiatrist.
7. Not all chronic pain patients have so-called "mental pain".
8. Not all chronic pain patients have "somatic pain".
9. Most of the pain patients are anxious.

10. Hesitate with knife, needle and drugs in the patients, suffering from a chronic pain syndrome.
11. Do not hesitate to use knife, needles and drugs, when dealing with patients, suffering from a malignant disease.
12. Humanity is the key of your success.

REFERENCES
1. Peter LJ, Hull R. 1976. The Peter Principle. London, Pan Books Ltd.
2. Sternbach, RA. 1968. Pain: A Psychophysiological Analysis. New York and London, Academic Press, Inc. Ltd.
3. Wall PD. 1979. Pain 6: 253-264.

REGIONAL BLOCKADE VERSUS ANALGESIC THERAPY

L. WIKLUND & G. ENGBERG

ABSTRACT

The early postoperative period is characterized by pain, high plasma catecholamine concentrations, increased energy expenditure, decreased arterial oxygen tension as well as increased glycogenolysis, lipolysis, proteolysis and low turn-over rate of glucose. Per- and postoperative local anaesthesia has often been supposed to counteract some of these phenomena without causing ventilatory depression or mental confusion. During the past few years a number of studies have been carried out in our department in order to elucidate possible differences between systemic analgesics and different local anaesthetic blockades. We have found that adequately performed local anaesthesia as well as systemic analgesic therapy relieve postoperative pain and decrease the increased total energy expenditure towards the normal range. An important difference is perhaps that local anaesthetic techniques during surgery results in a better maintenance of the body core temperature, resulting in less postoperative increase of the systemic oxygen uptake and less strain on the cardiovascular system. It also seems that less interference with ventilatory function is accomplished if local anaesthetic techniques are used. Thus, after orthopaedic surgery of the hip continuous epidural block results in a better oxygen delivery compared to systemic analgesics. It has, however, been difficult to demonstrate any reduction in the rate of respiratory complications. Only recently a large prospective clinical trial on postoperative intercostal blocks has shown a 50 % reduction in pulmonary complications after upper abdominal surgery. It has also been possible to show that local postoperative anaesthesia causes less mental confusion, less bowel problems and less thromboembolic disease.

For more than 10 years the Department of Anaesthesiology in Uppsala has been involved in studies of the physiological effects of general and orthopaedic surgery, anaesthesia and postoperative analgesic therapy. In our studies of postoperative analgesia, we have made comparisons between conventional centrally-acting analgesics administered intramuscularly on demand, and different regional blockades produced by local anaesthetic agents. Studies of regionally administered opiates are also in progress in our department, but the results will be presented elsewhere.

Physiological effects of anaesthesia and surgery

The postoperative period before administration of analgesic therapy is characterized by the following physiological features:
1. The systemic oxygen uptake is substantially increased (13, 5, 29, 38, 25) after operations under general anaesthesia. The increase is most pro-nounced during the first 12 h after surgery (13, 22); furthermore, it seems to be proportional to the trauma inflicted upon the patient (22) and the magnitude of the postoperative pain, and it is often more pro-nounced in younger patients than in older ones. The regional oxygen uptake in the leg (33) and the splanchnic area (38, 34) are also proportional to the increase in systemic oxygen uptake, while oxygen uptake by the human brain is on the same level as preoperatively. After operations under regional anaesthesia, the systemic oxygen uptake is not so greatly increased (25).
2. The systemic arterio-venous (a-v) oxygen difference seems to vary between normal and high values. The normal values are encountered after regional anaesthesia (e.g. epidural anaesthesia) and after general anaesthesia in young fit patients, while older patients have higher values, especially after general anaesthesia (38, 25). Large a-v oxygen differences are often found in patients suffering from cardiac disease.
3. After general anaesthesia, the arterial oxygen tension is reduced by some 15 %, while the arterial carbon dioxide tension remains fairly constant (27, 12, 5). The hypoxaemia after general anaesthesia is considered to be a consequence of a lowered functional residual capacity and ensuing closing of airways in dependent parts of the lungs (2, 28). In addition, micro-embolism of the lungs might play a role (24, 7). After surgery under regional anaesthesia, the arterial oxygen tension is better maintained (29, 25).

4. Surgery under general anaesthesia increases the mobilization of peripheral fat stores by lipolysis (39, 23, 33). In addition, hepatic glycogenolysis is enhanced and the peripheral utilization of glucose is decreased (34). The result is hyperglycaemia. Hepatic gluconeogenesis is also substantially increased (39). All these metabolic effects are believed to be mediated mainly through sympathetic nervous and circulating catecholamines as well as corticosteroids. Surgery under regional anaesthesia seems to have less pronounced metabolic effects, especially when intraoperative epidural anaesthesia is used which blocks the greater part of the thoracic sympathetic nervous system (15, 20). Certain metabolic effects, however, remain also after regional anaesthesia (9).

5. The physiological changes recorded intra- and postoperatively are believed to cause, or at least contribute to, postoperative complications such as thromboembolic disease and various respiratory problems. Depending on the method of diagnosis different incident rates of pulmonary complications have been recorded (40). Elective upper abdominal surgery thus carries a risk of 5 - 55 % of respiratory complications. Risk factors are old age, overweight, smoking and chronic bronchitis. Preoperative negative values of (FRC - CC) are closely connected to postoperative X-ray pulmonary abnormalities (42). Duration of general anaesthesia is also connected to the incidence of respiratory complications (41), while such a relation does not seem to exist for regional anaesthesia.

Physiological effects of postoperative analgesia
1. Systemic oxygen uptake

The postoperatively increased oxygen uptake may be reduced almost to the preoperative level by both regional blockades and centrally-acting conventional analgesics (38, 4). This may be illustrated by the finding that splanchnic blockade or intramuscularly administered opiates reduce energy expenditure (measured as systemic oxygen uptake) to the preoperative level, indicating that pain plays an extremely important role in the high energy expenditure in the early postoperative period (38). The finding also demonstrates that the systemic oxygen uptake may be almost unchanged immediately after surgery, provided that the patient is kept calm, free from pain and does not move around in bed (38, 4). The mediator of this increased energy expenditure has often been considered to be mediated by the sympathoadrenergic system, as measurements have shown high levels of catecholamines

(Stjernström et al., in preparation) and fatty acids and high blood levels of glycerol (39).

Recent studies in our department have, however,shown that the patients operated upon under general anaesthesia appear to have a decreased per-operative oxygen uptake resulting in lost energy content and an ensuing decrease in body heat, and furthermore, that the postoperative increase in energy expenditure is directly correlated to the peroperatively lost heat. As the oxygen uptake during surgery under epidural anaesthesia is maintained at the normal level, the postoperative energy expenditure is also very little increased (Henneberg et al., in preparation).

2. Arterio-venous oxygen difference

In general terms, it may be stated that the postoperative a-v oxygen difference is small in connection both with regional blockades and with centrally-acting analgesics in young patients (29, 31, 38, 25). Thus, both methods may cause a so-called hyperkinetic systemic circulation. However, as pointed out by Renck (29) from our department, the systemic a-v oxygen difference tends to be smaller during epidural blockades as compared to opiate analgesia on demand. This is true especially in elderly patients, who show fairly high cardiac output values and small systemic a-v oxygen differences in connection with postoperative thoracic and lumbar epidural blockade (29, 31, 38, 25). On the other hand, Modig (25) found that after administration of conventional intramuscular analgesics the elderly patient often had an increased a-v oxygen difference and a low mixed venous oxygen content, together with a reduced cardiac output. Clinically this sometimes resulted in a seriously low arterial oxygen tension, with cardiac arrhythmia such as atrial fibrillation, a finding which was never encountered in the group receiving lumbar epidural blockade.

3. Arterial oxygen tension

As mentioned above, arterial oxygen tension is lowered after general anaesthesia, especially in elderly patients who are given postoperative opiate analgesia on demand (27, 12, 5, 29, 31, 38, 25). Contrary to what was previously believed, it has been found that this is usually not due to decreased alveolar ventilation. Cardiac disease may, however, cause a hypokinetic circulation with a high a-v oxygen difference, which will result in a low arterial oxygen tension. More important, a reason for the hypoxaemia is the increased pulmonary shunting of venous blood after general anaesthesia and opiate postoperative analgesia (14, 25). This effect is not due to a true shunt, but to a pathological scatter of V/Q ratios which is created by airway closure in dependent parts of the lungs. Epidural blockade after total hip replacement promotes oxygenation as it does not alter the shunt or venous admixture (25). Similar positive effects on arterial oxygen tension were also noted by Sjögren & Wright (31) in connection with post-operative thoracic epidural blockade. In their study, however, this blockade also caused muscular weakness in the thoracic cage, with consequent failure in dynamic respiratory tests. Moreover, in a thorough investigation of pulmonary and chest wall mechanics (16, 17, 18) it was demonstrated that also intercostal blocks given to healthy volunteers caused some decrease in respiratory muscle strength in addition to a slight decrease in functional residual capacity (FRC). In a clinical series Engberg (11) found that uni-lateral intercostal blocks improved the arterial blood oxygenation after upper abdominal surgery under general anaesthesia. It was also demonstrated that this effect was achieved in parallel with some improvement of forced vital capacity, peak expiratory flow and forced expiratory volume. It seems reasonable to believe that the improvement of the spirometric variables was more related to the relief of pain and the bronchodilatation caused by the adrenaline added to the local anaesthetic solution (6), while the somewhat better arterial oxygen tension might be caused by a reduction in FRC and bronchodilatation.

4. It has been mentioned above that the early metabolic alterations after surgical trauma are believed to be mainly a result of pain and increased sympatho-adrenergic activity. These questions will be dealt with in more detail by Dr. Kehlet. I would only stress that neither opiate intramuscular analgesia nor splanchnic blockade (which also blocks the efferent nerve fibres to the adrenals) seems to alter the metabolic reaction to the surgical trauma, as evidenced by monitoring of the hepatic uptake or peripheral release of gluconeogenetic substrates (39, 34). As pointed out above thoracic epidural anaesthesia after abdominal surgery does not eliminate all metabolic effects of the surgical trauma (9).

5. Thromboembolic and pulmonary complications

General anaesthesia in connection with upper abdominal surgery frequently entails a high risk of different pulmonary complications (21, 36, 3, 1). Intraoperative nerve blockades have been found to reduce the incidence of these complications (10). Opinions have differed, however, concerning the beneficial effects of postoperative regional blockades (30, 8, 32, 37).

Pulmonary function as monitored by spirometry has generally not been
restored to the preoperative level (32, 31, 37, 16, 17, 18). There has also
been considerable doubt regarding the effects on postoperative lung complications. Findings in a recent extensive study (on about 400 patients)
in our department seem to shed some light on the problem (Engberg, in preparation). Thus, it was demonstrated that in patients who had undergone
cholecystectomy the incidence of pulmonary complications (radiologically
proven after clinical suspicion) was reduced from 12 to 6 % if the patients
were given a postoperative intercostal blockade. It was also noteworthy
that all the pulmonary complications after the blockades occurred in
patients over 60 years of age, while such complications also occurred in
younger patients when no intercostal block was given. In contrast, postoperative bilateral intercostal blockade had no effect on the incidence
of pulmonary complications after gastric resections and repair of
diaphragmatic hernias and in patients over 60 years of age, but the
complications were less severe and appeared later after surgery.

Thromboembolic disease constitutes a major problem after extensive
general and orthopaedic surgery. A large number of studies have shown that
often a majority of the patients suffer from deep venous thrombosis postoperatively (19). It was recently pointed out (26) that the incidence of
deep venous thrombosis after total hip replacement under general anaesthesia
combined with conventional opiate analgesia administered on demand was
73 %, as compared with 20 % for epidural blockade which was prolonged postoperatively. The incidence of pulmonary embolism was proportionally
diminished. Two principal mechanisms for this effect have been suggested,
and from recent observations they appear probable: firstly, the accelerated
leg blood flow after the sympathetic nervous block created by the epidural
blockade; and secondly, pharmacological effects on the balance between
clotting and fibrinolysis (26).

Up til now, I have deliberately left out the results of postoperative
interviews with patients concerning any painful experiences during the
course of analgesic treatment. I believe that the results of such investigations, or similar ones in which recordings are made of patients' requests
for additional analgesic treatment, may vary considerably and will quite
certainly be biased by the opinions and experience of the medical staff,
by the investigator and by the patient himself. It is considered that the
analgesic method practised with skill and experience after careful selection

for the individual patient and for the surgery concerned will prove to be the best in each situation. The final choice will be made in accordance with the experience and opinions of the anaesthesiologist. Thus, Engberg (1983) has demonstrated that intercostal blocks after cholecystectomies and choledocholithotomies considerably reduce the need for centrally-acting analgesics. On the other hand, the studies made by Tamsen (35) have shown that patient-controlled analgesic therapy (PACAT) might cause a similarly adequate analgesia well suited for the postoperative surgical patient.

Nevertheless, in our department we are convinced that an increasing number of our patients will gain most benefit from the use of methods based on careful regional blockades produced by regional anaesthetic techniques. These effects can be listed as follows:

Physiological   Less increase in oxygen uptake
                  Increased cardiac output
                  Improved ventilation
                  Decreased venous admixture
                  Improved arterial oxygenation

Clinical   Better and more constant analgesia
                  No central nervous depression
                  Often earlier mobilization
                  Earlier normalization of gastrointestinal function
                  Fewer pulmonary and thromboembolic complications

Disadvantages   Urinary retention
                  Sometimes muscular weakness

REFERENCES

1. Albert J, Löfström B, Pernow B. Postoperative pulmonary complications. Acta Chir Scand 129:395, 1964.
2. Alexander J I, Spence A A, Parikh R K, Stuart B. The role of airway closure in postoperative hypoxaemia. Brit J Anaesth 45:34, 1973.
3. Anscombe A. Pulmonary complications of abdominal surgery. Lloyd-Lube, London, 1957.
4. Arturson M G S. Metabolic changes following thermal injury. Wld J Surg 2:203, 1978.

5. Bay J, Nunn J F, Prys-Roberts C. Factors influencing arterial PO_2 during recovery from anaesthesia. Brit J Anaesth 40:398, 1968.
6. Bergh N P, Dottori O, Ax:son Löf B, Simonsson B G, Ygge H. Effect of intercostal block on lung function after thoracotomy. Acta Anaesth Scand Suppl 24:85, 1966.
7. Bowald S, Eriksson I, Wiklund L. The influence of heparin on haemodynamics and blood gases during abdominal aortic surgery. Acta Chir Scand 146:333, 1979.
8. Bromage P R. Extradural analgesia for pain relief. Brit J Anaesth 39:721, 1967.
9. Buckley F P, Kehlet H, Brown N S, Scott D B. Postoperative glucose tolerance during extradural analgesia. Brit J Anaesth 54:325, 1982.
10. Dripps R D, van Deming M. Postoperative atelectasis and pneumonia. Diagnosis, etiology and management based upon 1240 cases of upper abdominal surgery. Ann Surg 124:94, 1946.
11. Engberg G. Single-dose intercostal nerve blocks with etidocaine for pain relief after upper abdominal surgery. Acta Anaesth Scand Suppl 60:43, 1975.
12. Georg J, Hornum I, Mellengaard K. The mechanism of hypoxaemia after laparotomy. Thorax 22:382, 1967.
13. Harild S. Untersuchungen über die postoperativen Veränderungen des Minutenvolumes des Herzens. Arch Klin Chir 201:249, 1941.
14. Hollmén A, Saukkonen J. The effects of postoperative epidural analgesia versus centrally acting opiate on physiological shunt after upper abdominal operation. Acta Anaesth Scand 16:147, 1972.
15. Hume D M, Egdahl R H. The importance of the brain in the endocrine response to injury. Am Surg 150:697, 1959.
16. Jakobson S, Ivarsson I. Effects of intercostal nerve blocks (Etidocaine 0.5 %) on chest wall mechanics in cholecystectomized patients. Acta Anaesth Scand 21:497, 1977.
17. Jakobson S, Ivarsson I. Effects of intercostal nerve blocks (bupivacaine 0.25 % and etidocaine 0.5 %) on chest wall mechanics in healthy men. Acta Anaesth Scand 21:489, 1977.
18. Jakobson S, Fridriksson H, Hedenström H, Ivarsson I. Effects of intercostal nerve blocks on pulmonary mechanics in healthy men. Acta Anaesth Scand 24:482, 1980.
19. Kakkar V V. Deep-vein thrombosis: Detection and prevention. Circulation 51:8, 1975.
20. Kehlet H, Brandt M R, Rem J. Role of neurogenic stimuli in mediating the endocrine-metabolic response to surgery. J Parent Ent Nutr 4:152, 1980.
21. King D S. Postoperative pulmonary complications. A statistical study based upon two years personal observation. Surg Gynec Obstet 56:43, 1933.
22. Kinney J M, Long C L, Duke J H. Carbohydrate and nitrogen metabolism after injury. Energy Metabolism in Trauma, ed. R Porter & J Knight, J & A Churchill, London, pp 103-126, 1970.
23. Knitza R, Clasen R, Theiss D, Lanz E. Veränderungen im Kohlenhydrat- und Fettstoffwechsel unter Spinal- bzw. Neuroleptanaesthesie und Operation. Anaesthesist 28:63, 1979.
24. Lahnborg G, Lagergren H, Hedenstierna G. Effect of low-dose heparin prophylaxis on arterial oxygen tension after high laparotomy. Lancet i:54, 1976.

25. Modig J. Respiration and circulation after total hip replacement surgery. Acta Anaesth Scand 20:225, 1976.
26. Modig J, Borg T, Karlström G, Maripuu E, Sahlstedt B. Thromboembolism after total hip replacement: Role of epidural and general anesthesia. Anesth Analg 62:174, 1983.
27. Nunn J F. Hypoxaemia after general anaesthesia. Lancet ii:631, 1962.
28. Rehder K, Marsh H M, Rodarte J R, Hyatt R E. Airway closure. Anesthesiology 47:40, 1977.
29. Renck H. The elderly patient after anaesthesia and surgery. Acta Anaesth Scand Suppl 34, 1969.
30. Simpson B R, Parkhouse J, Marshall R, Lambrects W. Extradural analgesia and the prevention of postoperative respiratory complications. Brit J Anaesth 33:628, 1961.
31. Sjögren S, Wright B. Circulation, respiration and lidocaine concentration during continuous epidural blockade. Acta Anaesth Scand Suppl 46, 1972.
32. Spence A A, Smith G. Post-operative analgesia and lung function. A comparison of morphine and extradural block. Brit J Anaesth 43:144, 1971.
33. Stjernström H, Jorfeldt L, Wiklund L. Influence of abdominal surgical trauma upon the turnover of some blood-borne energy metabolites in the human leg. J Parent Ent Nutr 5:207, 1981.
34. Stjernström H, Jorfeldt L, Wiklund L. Interrelationship between splanchnic and leg exchange of glucose and other blood-borne energy metabolites during abdominal surgical trauma. Clin Physiol 1:59, 1981.
35. Tamsen A, Hartvig P, Fagerlund C, Dahlström B, Bondesson U. Patient-controlled analgesic therapy: Clinical experience. Acta Anaesth Scand Suppl 74:157, 1982.
36. Thorén L. Postoperative pulmonary complications. Observation on their prevention by means of physiotherapy. Acta Chir Scand 107:193, 1954.
37. Wahba W M, Don H F, Craig D B. Postoperative epidural analgesia: Effects on lung volumes. Canad Anaesth Soc J 22:519, 1975.
38. Wiklund L. Splanchnic oxygen uptake in relation to systemic oxygen uptake during postoperative splanchnic blockade and postoperative fentanyl analgesia. Acta Anaesth Scand Suppl 58:29, 1975.
39. Wiklund L, Jorfeldt L. Effects of abdominal surgery under general anaesthesia and of postoperative analgesic therapy on splanchnic exchange of some blood-borne energy metabolites. Acta Anaesth Scand Suppl 58:41, 1975.
40. Wirén J E, Janzon L, Hellekant C. Respiratory complications after upper abdominal surgery. Acta Chir Scand 147:623, 1981.
41. Wirén J E, Janzon L. Risk factors for postoperative respiratory complications and their predictive value. Acta Chir Scand 148:479, 1982.
42. Wirén J E, Lindell S E, Hellekant C. Pre- and postoperative lung function in the sitting and supine position related to postoperative chest X-ray abnormalities and arterial hypoxemia. Clin Physiol 3:257, 1983.

ANALGESIC AND RESPIRATORY EFFECTS OF SUBCUTANEOUS AND
EPIDURALLY ADMINISTERED MORPHINE IN RATS

ROB H.W.M. VAN DEN HOOGEN

SUMMARY

The experiments presented here examined the in vivo analgesic
and respiratory effects of morphine after epidural and
subcutaneous administration in rats.
Both subcutaneous and epidural injections of morphine exerted
dose-dependent analgesic effects. Analgesic effects measured
in the tail flick test were biphasic. Both subcutaneous and
epidural morphine produced dose-dependent respiratory
depressant effects expressed by a decrease in the slope of
the carbondioxide response curve.
Respiratory depression at the time of analgesic peak effect
at equi-analgesic dosages of morphine was more pronounced
after subcutaneous administration than after epidural administration.

INTRODUCTION

The principal use of morphine and morphine-like drugs derives
from their ability to relieve pain.
When used as an analgesic, opiates may produce a variety of
additional effects including miosis, nausea, vomiting, inhibition of peristalsis, sedation and respiratory depression.[1]
Respiratory depression is prominent among these additional
effects; even after epidural administration this is life
threatening and limits the use of opiates in the treatment of
acute and chronic pain. There is a need for the characteriza-
tion of opiate respiratory effect in animals relative to
their analgesic action. In order to study these two phenomena
animal conditions in both series of experiments must be
comparable. Analgesics have been studied extensively in
otherwise intact animals using techniques such as the hot
plate and tail withdrawal test.
Opiate respiratory depressant effects must be studied with
regards to frequency and tidal volume respectively while
breathing air and the reaction to an increase in inspiratory
carbondioxide on these parameters.
In order to investigate these respiratory effects it is
necessary to use a method which permits measurements without
the use of anaesthetic drugs, except for the one to investigate, which themselves effect respiration. For the same
reason it is essential not to restrain or thracheostomize the
animal. In this series of experiments whole body plethysmo-

graphy was used to determine carbondioxide response curves with the steady state method.

MATERIALS AND METHODS

Animals
Subjects were male Wistar rats of 250-300 g.
They were housed individually in standard rodent cages with free access to food and water. All animals were used only once in experiments.

Measurement of analgesia
Latency for tail withdrawal[2] after immersion of the tail in a 55°C water bath was measured to the nearest 0.1 sec with a cut off time of 30 sec to avoid damage to the tail.

Measurement of respiration
Steady state respiration in rats breathing air of different percentages of carbondioxide in air (4-6-8%) was measured by means of a modification[3] of the whole body plethysmographic technique described by Drorbaugh and Fenn.[4] This technique has been published in detail elsewhere.[5] The slopes of the carbondioxide response curves at the time of analgesic peak effect after subcutaneous administration, and the least slopes in the first four hours after epidural administration were used for data analysis.

Epidural catheterization
For the epidural administration rats under Thalamonal[R] and pentobarbital anaesthesia were implanted with an epidural catheter via a drilled hole in the fourth lumbar vertebra. The catheter was subcutaneously tunneled towards the neck region.[6]
Rats were allowed to recover one week from surgery before they were used in experiments.

Drugs
For subcutaneous administration doses of freshly dissolved morphine (0.16, 0.63, 2.5, 10, 40 and 160 mg kg^{-1}) were injected in a volume of 10 ml kg^{-1}.
For epidural administration doses of freshly dissolved morphine (0.16, 0.63, 2.5, 10 and 40 µg rat^{-1}) were injected in a volume of 20 µl.

RESULTS

Analgesic effects
The dose relation between increasing doses of morphine, both after subcutaneous or epidural administration, and the median peak latency in the tail flick test of 9 animals per concentration of morphine was biphasic (fig. 1). The computed equi-analgesic D10" dose, the dose of morphine needed to achieve a latency of 10 sec in the tail flick test, was found to be 5.3 mg kg^{-1} for subcutaneous administration and 2.9 µg rat^{-1} for epidural administration respectively.

Respiratory effects
Subcutaneous administered morphine (0-40 mg kg^{-1}) had no significant effect on the frequency of breathing while rats were breathing air. Only the dose 160 mg kg^{-1} showed a slight

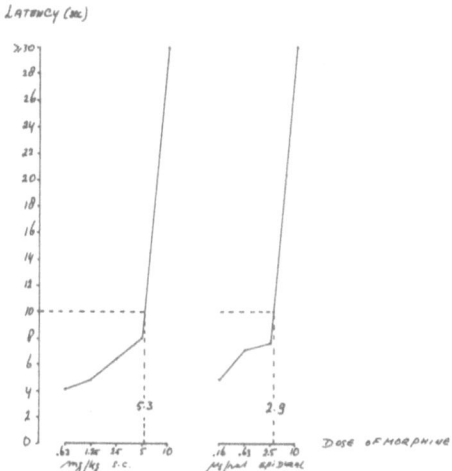

Fig. 1 Latency in the tail flick test in seconds on the ordinate and increasing dose of morphine, mg kg^{-1} for subcutaneous and μg rat^{-1} for epidural administration, on the abscissa. Each data point represents the median peak latency of 9 animals per concentration. Equi-analgesic Dl0" doses were computed by the linear regression method.

decrease in frequency. But breathing 8% carbondioxide in air produced an almost linear decrease in frequency on increasing doses of morphine (fig. 2).
Subcutaneous administered morphine (0-40 mg kg^{-1}) produced a dose related decrease in tidal volume while breathing air. But the highest dose (160 mg kg^{-1}) increased tidal volume. This effect was again more pronounced while animals were breathing 8% carbondioxide in air (fig. 3).
With frequency and tidal volume minute volume of breathing was computed and corrected for body weight.
The effects of increasing doses of s.c. morphine on VE are summarized in fig. 4.
From 0 to 10 mg kg^{-1} there was no significant difference while breathing air; 40 and 160 mg kg^{-1} decreased VE to the same level. Breathing 8% CO_2 in air, there was no significant difference in minute volume from 0 to 0.63 mg kg^{-1} morphine, then VE decreased to 60 ml min^{-1} 100 g^{-1} at the level of 40 mg kg^{-1} and then became stationary due to the increase in tidal volume. The regression lines of the carbondioxide response curves on VE were computed by the least square method. These regression lines and their corresponding slopes which reflect respiratory depression are shown in fig. 5.

222

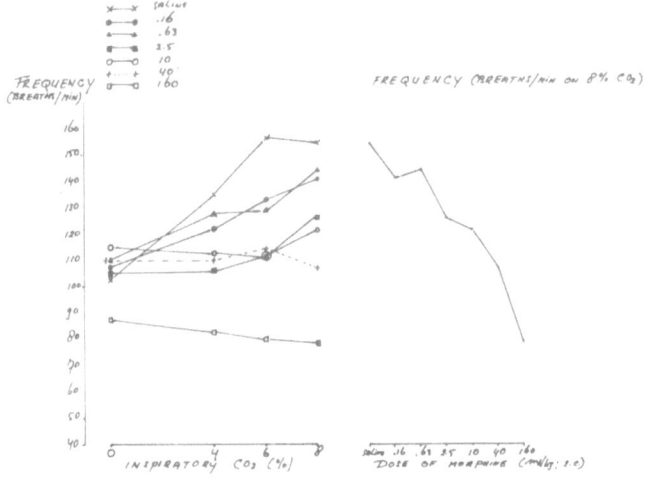

Fig. 2   Frequency of breathing (breath min^{-1}) on the ordinate
and percentage inspiratory carbondioxide on the
abscissa. Doses of s.c. morphine are in top of the
figure. Each data point represents the mean frequency
of 5 animals. On the right side the effect of 8% CO_2
in air on frequency of breathing for the different
doses of s.c. morphine.

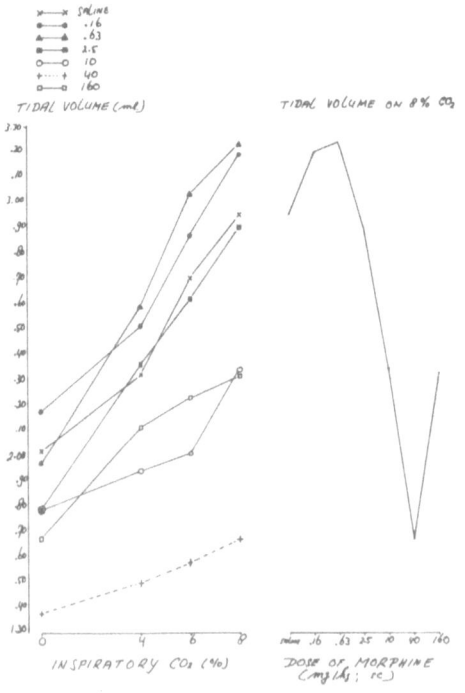

Fig. 3   Tidal volume (ml) on the ordinate against percentage
inspiratory carbondioxide on the abscissa. On the
right side the effect of 8% CO_2 in air on tidal
volume for the different doses of s.c. morphine.

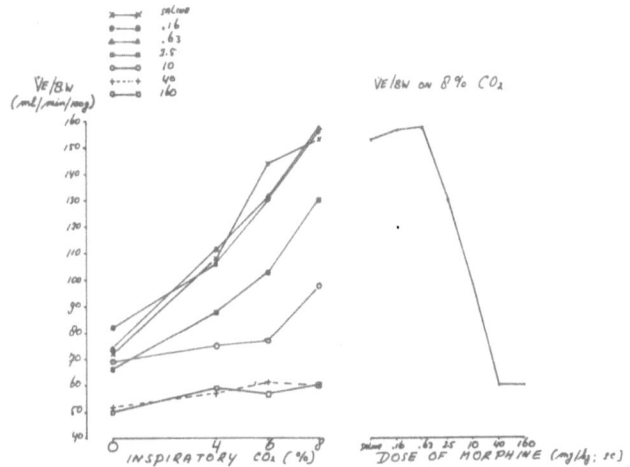

Fig. 4   Minute volume of breathing corrected for body weight
(ml min^{-1} 100 g^{-1}) on the ordinate against percentage
inspiratory carbondioxide on the abscissa. On the
right side the effect of 8% CO_2 in air on VE/BW for
the different doses of s.c. morphine.

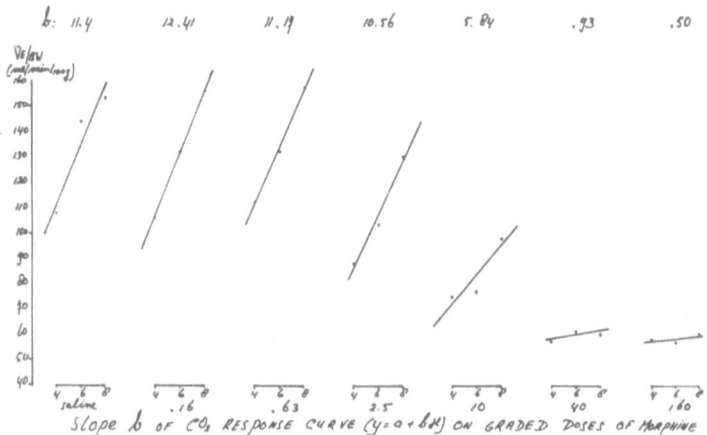

Fig. 5   Slope b of CO_2 response curve (y = a + bH) on graded
doses of morphine.

The same series of calculations were carried out for epidural
administered morphine (data not shown here).
The slopes of the carbondioxide response curve per concentration of morphine both after subcutaneous and epidural administration are put together in fig. 6.

224

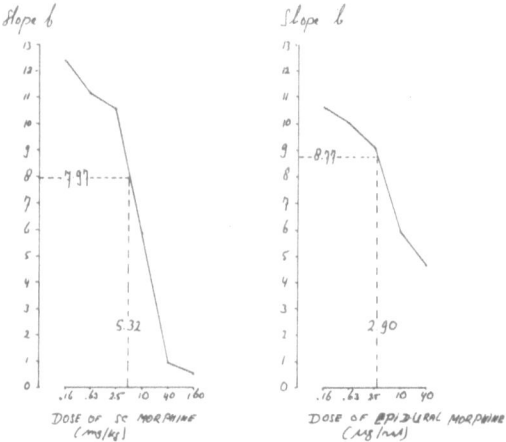

Fig. 6 Slope b of the carbondioxide response curve on the
        ordinate and increasing dose of morphine on the
        abscissa. The computed slopes at equi-analgesic D10
        dose are drawn in.

The computed slope at equi-analgesic dose (the so called D10
dose) was found to be 7.97 and 8.77 for subcutaneous and
epidural administration respectively.
For further evaluation of this only small difference we
computed the slopes for two, four and eight times the equi-
analgesic dose, by the method of linear regression, for both
ways of administration.
As demonstrated in fig. 7 on increasing levels of analgesia
epidural administered morphine produced less respiratory
depression than after subcutaneous administration.

CONCLUSION

A sensitive measure for the detection of respiratory
depression is a change in the slope of the carbondioxide
response curve of unrestrained, unanaesthetized animals.
As demonstrated here frequency of breathing while breathing
air is not a valid parameter for the detection of respiratory
depression in rats.
Morphine both after subcutaneous and epidural administration
causes a respiratory depression in rats, which is less
pronounced after epidural administration on increasing levels
of analgesia. Both after s.c. and epidural administration
respiratory depression occurs at the lowest dose which
produces analgesia.
After subcutaneous administration the time of analgesic peak
effect corresponds with the time of peak effect of
respiratory depression (van den Hoogen, unpublished data),

but after epidural administration the peak effect of respiratory depression occurred later than the peak time of analgesia with large individual differences (1-4 hour).

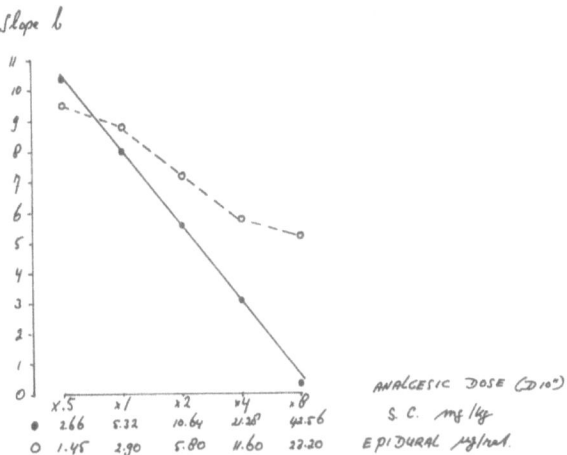

Fig. 7   Slope b of the carbondioxide response curve on the ordinate and 0.5, 1, 2, 4 and 8 times the equianalgesic D10" dose of s.c. and epidural morphine respectively. Slopes for the different doses were computed with linear regression.

REFERENCES

1. Goodman LS and Gilman A: The Pharmacological Basis of Therapeutics

2. Janssen PAJ, Niemegeers CJE: Arzneimittel Forsch. 13, 502-507, 1963

3. Bartlett D Jr., and Tenney SM: Resp. Physiol. 10, 384-395, 1970

4. Drorbaugh JE and Fenn WO: Pediatrics 16, 81-87, 1955

5. Colpaert FC and van den Hoogen RHWM: Life Sciences 33, 1065-1073, 1983

6. Van den Hoogen RHWM and Colpaert FC: Pharmac. Biochem. Behav. 15 (3), 515-516, 1981

CONTINUOUS EPIDURAL ANAESTHESIA
ADVANTAGES AND DISADVANTAGES

M. D'A. STANTON-HICKS

As a technique, continuous epidural analgesia has been available since the introduction of catheters small enough to pass through introducing needles. The most commonly employed for this purpose was originally designed by Tuohy to facilitate the passage of a catheter into the sub-arachnoid space for continuous spinal block.[1]

Initially, the short-acting amide local anaesthetics, like lignocaine were employed, either as a continuous infusion delivered as a drip by gravity, or by infusion pump.[2,3,4] Unfortunately, because of the short duration of action of these agents, a high dose rate was necessary to provide adequate analgesia and this, in turn, was then responsible for un-acceptably high local anaesthetic blood levels.[5] Clinically these would be manifested by drowsiness, cardiovascular depression and rarely, pre-ictal signs such as **nystagmus** and involuntary muscle twitching. With the advent of the long-acting local anaesthetic bupivacaine, most of these problems vanished, although when the technique was prolonged beyond the second postoperative day, tachyphylaxis already a nuisance with the short-acting agents, also becomes evident. While the acute tolerance which occurs with these long-acting local anaesthetics develops more slowly, it is nevertheless responsible for some of the difficulties which are associ-ated with the technique of continuous epidural analgesia that will be discussed here.

As an alternative to conventional methods of providing pain relief after surgery, continuous epidural analgesia serves two purposes. Firstly, the relief of pain, and secondly, the preservation of function. While the former would seem obvious and is the natural extension of that analgesia provided during surgery, the preservation of function refers to the prevention of any circumstances which would impair respiratory, cardiovascular or alimentary function. It is for this particular aspect that epidural analgesia is proposed as an alternative to the parenteral administration of narcotic analgesics which at best relieve much of the surgical pain, provide some sedation but do so at the expense of respiratory and cardiovascular depression, and may in fact promote ileus.

Many of the secondary gains which accrue from epidural analgesia are due to the sympathectomy, the block of visceral afferent nerves, and the influence of the unopposed vagus on bowel function. The beneficial effects of postoperative epidural analgesia are summarized in Figure 1. See appendix.

Let us consider pain first, unlike most other analgesics which derive their effects through a central action, conduction anaesthesia by definition, blocks segmentally the nociceptive input to the spinal cord, which in turn prevents its onward transmission and perception as pain. Pharmacologically this approach has the advantage over parenteral analgesia of being both economical and specific. In addition, because the relief of pain is almost, if not complete, because both visceral and somatic components are blocked, it becomes possible in selected cases to mobilize those high risk patients, even on the evening of their surgery, without causing them pain. The obese postcholecystectomy patient with a predisposition to thromboembolic disease would fit this category of patient. In addition, such a patient, together with others having upper abdominal surgery, develop a high incidence of pulmonary atelectasis which in some cases can lead on to hypostatic inflammatory conditions unless vigorous physical therapy is carried out.

A number of prospective studies have clearly demonstrated an improvement in respiratory function that accompanies segmental epidural blocks. This improvement is gained in spite of the obvious weakness of the intercostal and abdominal muscles. This weakness does impair the ability to cough, although not enough to prevent the expulsion of secretions. Certainly the difference in the expulsive effort caused by pain, and that due to the segmental motor block, greatly favours the use of the latter method of pain control. The vital capacity, severely impaired after abdominal surgery may, under the influence of segmental epidural block, be returned to seventy five percent of its preoperative value.[6] This fact has been referred to by Bromage as the Respiratory Restoration Factor (R.R.F.). Another physiological parameter which is improved by epidural block is the respiratory capacity which is a reflection of the improved chest compliance and is manifested both in quiet or deep breathing. Several authors have substantiated the improvement in the arterial oxygen and in the alveolar arterial oxygen difference which can be obtained by epidural block in postoperative patients.

Block of the sympathetic outflow, as already mentioned, is responsible for many of the beneficial changes of a functional nature which are associated with postoperative epidural analgesia. There are a number of surgical procedures which are associated with a high incidence of thromboembolic phenonomena. These are listed in the following table.

TABLE 1

Major prosthetic vascular surgery
Intrapelvic surgery
Surgery of the hip joint

Although it has been clearly shown experimentally that the lesion initiating the thrombus in the calf and pelvic veins commences during surgery, the prophylactic benefits of epidural analgesia continue into the postoperative period.[7,8]

The sympathetic disturbance which is a natural sequal to major prosthetic vascular surgery is inhibited if the conduction anaesthetic is continued into the postoperative period, with the result that clotting in the grafted segment is inhibited and spasm with extension of the thrombotic process is prevented downstream from the graft.[9] A number of well controlled studies have demonstrated the influence this technique has had on the re-operation rate after vascular surgery.[10]

Block of visceral afferent fibres which mediate pain from intra abdominal and pelvic surgery also interrupts nervous pathways mediating reflex effects from the segmental area of distribution. Adverse effects on the cardiovascular system in susceptible individuals can be avoided or minimized by preventing these reflexes by continuous epidural blocks. It is well recognized that postoperative pain through sympathetic stimulation can be responsible for further ischaemic injury in individuals with severe myocardial disease. Although there are still no statistically significant prospective studies which confirm the protective effect of epidural anaesthesia in such individuals, there is experimental evidence to support the benefits of sympathectomy on the ischaemic myocardium. So at least there would appear to be empiric reasons for recommending the use of continuous epidural analgesia for postoperative pain in patients with a history of ischaemic myocardial disease.

Finally, work during the past twenty years,[11,12,13] has shown that the stress response to surgery, particularly that in the lower abdomen and pelvis, is modified or inhibited if the level of analgesia is kept above T5. The catecholamine and cortisol levels which are normally elevated during and after surgery remain within preoperative values or are only

slightly raised during continuous epidural block. As a result, blood
sugar, renin and angiotensin levels are normal, at least during the first
24 postoperative hours.[14] By anticipating these effects of surgical trauma
with conduction analgesia, the organism is maintained in an anabolic state
rather than the characteristic post surgical catabolic phase. It is very
difficult to evaluate whether this modification of the neuroendocrine
response to surgery is beneficial in the long run. That the **net result**
is to the patient's advantage is provided by one study which showed that
there was a particularly reduced hospital confinement by patients who
were managed by continuous epidural block, compared with a comparable
group who had received general anaesthesia and postoperative narcotic administration.[15]

Following upper abdominal surgery, the modification of the stress
response by epidural block is greatly reduced, possibly because many
visceral afferents which travel via the vagus nerves are unaffected by
the block.

Having presented the reasons for advocating postoperative epidural
analgesia, we must now consider the disadvantages of the technique of
which, although surmountable, there are many. These are listed in order
of importance in Table 2.

TABLE 2

Logistics of providing epidural service
Cost
Training of personnel
Tachyphylaxis
Hypotension
Urinary retention

The logistics of providing an epidural service depend on many factors,
the most important being the time available which an anaesthetic department can allow for such activity. Obviously the resolve and interest of

individual anaesthesiologists is an essential ingredient, but would be of
little consequence unless the department can underwrite the time outside
of the provision of anaesthesia to enable such a service to be developed
in a hospital. A corollary to the development of an epidural service is
the training of nursing staff in the management of patients who are
receiving this form of analgesia. If one assumes that reinjection of
epidural catheters remains a physician's responsibility, at least it would
appear to be so in the foreseeable future, then for its success, a system
must be developed that will permit notification of the onset of a patient's
pain and an appropriately rapid response by the anaesthesia department to
reinject the catheter. If catheters are to be serviced on a reinjection
basis rather than by continuous infusion, the onset of tachyphylaxis can
only be delayed when the interval between the recrudescence of pain and
its response by reinjection are kept as short as possible, ideally within
30 minutes.[16] To facilitate such a response it would be appropriate to
assemble all patients with epidural catheters in a postoperative ward in
proximity to the operating theatre suite. This question becomes even
pertinent when one considers the use of intraepidural narcotics, although
I will confine my remarks here to the use of local anaesthetics only.

The question of hypotension is more theoretical than real. Certainly
the degree to which the blood pressure may fall following injection will
depend to some extent on the number of spinal segments blocked. However,
more important is the state of hydration of the patient. In practice
hypotension is not a real problem and one can expect falls in pressure of
no more than 10 percent mean arterial pressure in most cases. Also, if
the pressure falls, it will do so immediately following reinjection.

Urinary retention, common after all anaesthetics, occurs more frequently
after conduction anaesthesia. It is more common in males and in some

232

cases certainly requires catheterization, although the majority of patients can either void spontaneously or the nature of their surgery has already dictated the placement of urinary drainage.

Toxicity of local anaesthetics, unless they are placed directly into a blood vessel, is usually not a problem, even during the third or fourth postoperative days when tachyphylaxis has made it necessary to keep increasing the dose. The amount of local anaesthetic required in any 24 hour period with the intermittent injection technique is some 5 times less than that which would be required by the continuous infusion technique, which is another reason for commending this technique over the other. The features of the intermittent injection technique are summarized in Table 3.

TABLE 3

Lower total 24 hour dose
Lower toxicity
Better analgesia
Less tachyphylaxis
Labour intensive
Less hypotension
Less urinary retention

The purpose behind a continuous infusion epidural technique is an attempt to strike an equilibrium between the kinetics of uptake and distribution of local anaesthetic from the epidural space, such that the number of blocked spinal segments remains constant throughout the course of the infusion. That this is an ideal case is obvious since many perturbations of this attempted status quo like changing cardiovascular dynamics, diurnal metabolic fluctuations as well as acute local anaesthetic tolerance, can each singly or together alter the dose per segment requirements.

However these aspects notwithstanding, it is possible to utilize the

technique to advantage and spare the otherwise close supervision needed
to service the intermittent epidural technique.

As already mentioned, a higher dose of local anaesthetic is required
during any 24 hour period. The potential toxicity is, therefore, greater
compared with the intermittent technique. Because of the larger dose
used, tachyphylaxis tends to develop more rapidly. The risk of hypertension is greater since, if the dose rate is set too high, the segmental
level may ascend during the night, a time when the nursing supervision
is not as close as it might otherwise be. Conversely, if the infusion
rate is inadequate to maintain the desired segmental level, it will be
necessary to give a bolus injection in order to reestablish analgesia in
the desired segments. The characteristics of the continuous infusion
technique are summarized in Table 4.

TABLE 4

High total 24 hour dose
Potential higher toxicity
Poorer analgesia
Faster onset of tachyphylaxis
Infrequent servicing - less manpower
Greater risk of hypotension
More urinary retention

Whether a continuous infusion or intermittent technique is utilized,
the principal disadvantages relating to the staffing of such a service
and the most appropriate site remain in most institutions. Philosophically,
the cost, as it relates to the provision of an adequate manpower to run
such a service, should be surmountable. The case for this type of analgesia
is strong and if the functional aspects can be substantiated by well
controlled studies, there should be a cost benefit to the institution by
significantly reduced hospitalization times. The provision of space for
a postoperative ward may, in most existing institutions, be difficult to
find. The cost of placing such patients in a postoperative recovery unit,

at least in the United States, would be prohibitive. Likewise, it is
inappropriate to place routine post surgical patients in an intensive
care unit which is staffed and equipped to deal with patients requiring
multisystems support. It is equally difficult to contemplate placing
patients having continuous epidural analgesia on various surgical stations
throughout the hospital as it makes the servicing of such patients by
anaesthesia personnel a nightmare. Yet, at the present time one is faced
with this particular situation.

It would seem that the solution probably lies in our hands. If, as
I have tried to show, the advantages of this method of analgesia out-
weigh the disadvantages, most of which are circumstantial and logistic,
then we as anaesthesiologists need to make a case in support of those
criteria which would make this technique feasible. This argument must
be brought before such bodies as hospital planners and administrators.

A comparison of the current bed cost of patient care in a private
room, postoperative recovery room, intensive care unit and a hypothetical
postoperative ward ("old Victorian ward"), is shown in Figure 2. The
comparison is not odious and clearly illustrates and supports any
argument in defense of having such a facility in proximity to the department which would provide such a service.

APPENDIX
Figure 1 - Advantages of Epidural Block

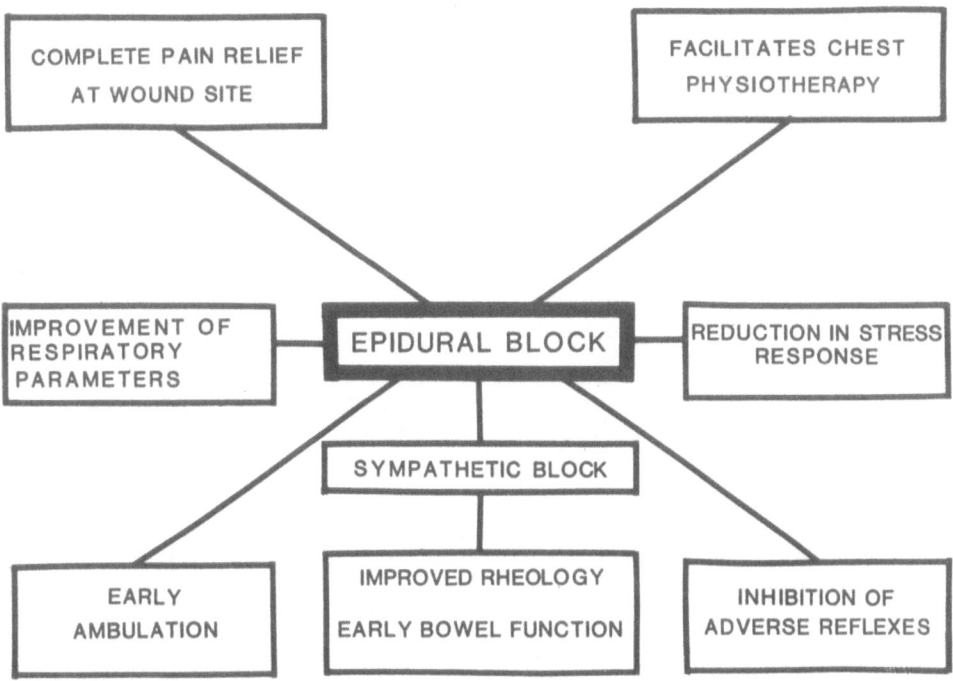

Figure 2

PRICE OF SURVEILLANCE IN USA, 1983

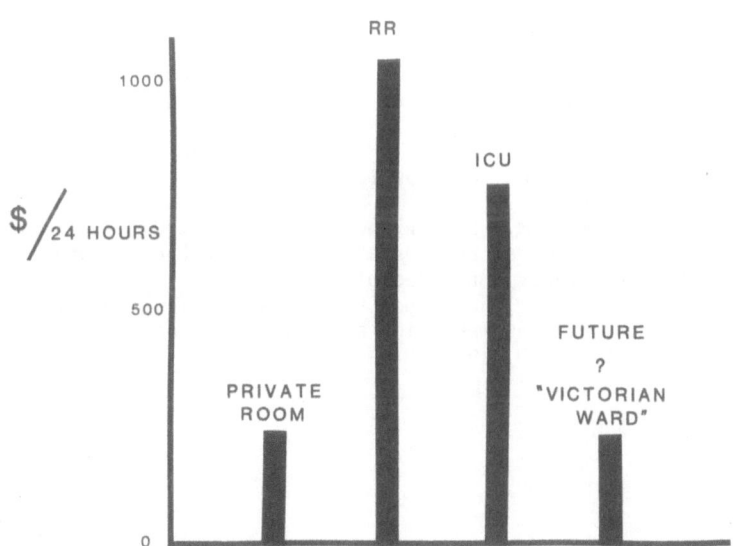

236

REFERENCES

1. Tuohy, E.B. Continuous Spinal Anesthesia: Its usefulness and technic involved. Anesthesiology 5:142, 1944
2. Griffiths, D.P.G., Diamond, A.W. and Cameron, J.D. Postoperative extradural analgesia following thoracic surgery. A feasibility study. Br. J. Anaesth. 47:48, 1975
3. Spoerel, W.E., Thomas, A., and Gerula, G.R. Continuous epidural analgesia: Experience with mechanical injection devices. Can. Anaes. Soc. J. 17:37, 1970
4. Green, R., and Dawkins, C.J.M. Postoperative analgesia: The use of continuous drip epidural block. Anaesthesia 21:372, 1966
5. Tucker, G.T., et al: Observed and predicted accumulation of local anaesthetic agents during continuous extradural analgesia. Br. J. Anaesth. 49:237, 1977
6. Bromage, P.R., Spirometry in assessment of analgesia after upper abdominal surgery: A method of comparing analgesic drugs. Br. Med. J., 2:589, 1955
7. Lahnborg, G. and Bergstrom, K. Clinical and haemostatic parameters related to thromboembolism and low-dose heparin prophylaxis in major surgery. Acta Clin. Scand. 141:590, 1975
8. Modig, J., Borg, T., Karlstrom, G., Maripui, E., Sahlstedt, B. Thromboembolism after hip replacement: role of epidural and of general anaesthesia. Anesth. Analg. 1982 (In press)
9. Sandman, W., Kremer, K., Wüst, H., Florack, G., Ruf, S. Funktions-kontrolle von rekonstruierten arterien durch postoperative elektromagnetische strömungsmessung. Thoraxchirurgie 25:427, 1977
10. Sandman, W., Wüst, H., Lerut, J. Der einfluss der periduralanaesthesie auf das strömungsverhalten in der vena femoraus. Neueaspekte in der regionalanaesthesie 2. Anaesthesiologie u intensivmedizin 138:128, 1981
11. Engquist, A., Brandt, M.R., Fernandes, A., Kehlet, H. The blocking effect of epidural analgesia on the adrenocortical and hyperglycenic responses to surgery. Acta Anaesthesiol. Scand. 21:330, 1977
12. Engquist, A., Fog-Møller, F., Christiansen, C., Thode, J., Vester-Anderson, T., Nistrup Madsen, S. Influence of epidural analgesia on the catecholamine and cyclic AMP responses to surgery. Acta Anaesthesia Scand. 24:17, 1980
13. Kehlet, H. The modifying effect of general and regional anesthesia on the endocrine-metabolic response to surgery. Regional Anesthesia. Supp. Vol. 7 4:38, 1982
14. Brandt, M.R., Ølgaard, K., Kehlet, H. Epidural analgesia inhibits the renin and aldosterone response to surgery. Acta Anaesthesiol. Scand. 23:267, 1979
15. Pflug, A.E., Murphy, T.M., Butler, S.H. and Tucker, G.T. The effects of postoperative peridural analgesia on pulmonary therapy and pulmonary complications. Anesthesiology 41:8, 1974
16. Bromage, P.R., Pettigrew, R.T. and Crowell, D.E. Tachyphylaxis in epidural analgesia 1. Augmentation and decay of local analgesia. J. Clin. Pharmacol. 9:30, 1969

THE ENDOCRINE-METABOLIC RESPONSE TO POSTOPERATIVE PAIN

H. Kehlet, N.C. Hjortsø and D. Bigler

Surgery represents a noxious stimulus to which the body reacts with both a local inflammatory response and a general response. The general response is characterized by profound endocrine changes leading to increased energy consumption and a shift in flow of substrates from storage to central organs. Although we still have no good explanation for this stress-response to injury, an improved understanding of the physiological changes resulting from anaesthesia and surgery has led to a reduction in postoperative morbidity during the last decades. Concomitantly, there has been an increased interest in techniques which may modify the endocrine-metabolic response to surgery, based upon the hypothesis that a reduction in the physiological changes to injury may also lead to a reduction in various aspects of postoperative morbidity. Diminishment of the trauma response presupposes understanding of the involved release mechanisms, including the relative role of afferent neurogenic stimuli, humoral substances released from the wound, pain stimuli, the influence of heat loss, hypoxemia, hypovolemia, psychological factors etc.[1].

This review is a short summary on the influence of pain per se on the postoperative endocrine-metabolic response and the modification of the stress-response as a result of pain alleviation by current available techniques. For a more detailed information the reader is referred to a recent review[2].

INFLUENCE OF PAIN PER SE ON ENDOCRINE-METABOLIC
PARAMETERS.

Surprisingly little information is available, but in
patients with chronic non-surgical pain nitrogen balance was
more negative during days with pain compared to days without
pain and nitrogen balance improved after administration of
analgesics with subsequent alleviation of pain[3]. Experimental pain during sustained isometric muscle contraction during
ischemia led to an increase in plasma cortisol but not in
various plasma endorphins[4].

THE INFLUENCE OF POSTOPERATIVE PAIN ON ENDOCRINE-
METABOLIC CHANGES.

During recent years basic research on the mechanisms by
which noxious stimuli are processed in the central nervous
system has led to an improved understanding of pain and
treatment of pain[5, 6, 7]. Peripheral mediation of pain
following a noxious stimulus involves local release of endo-
genous algesic substances such as histamine, serotonin,
kinins and potassium, which all may excite the afferent
neurogenic fibers directly. Furthermore, the release of
prostaglandins and substance-P may alter microcirculation
and permeability thereby sensitizing the nerve terminals for
transmission of the noxious stimulus. The centripetal transmission of pain stimuli goes predominantly through C- and
Aδ-fibers into the dorsal horn where the primary transmitters are substance-P, and probably glutamic acid, VIP,
CCK and somatostatin. The further rostrad transmission of
pain stimuli from the dorsal horn may be modified by
descending pathways from the cerebrum using serotonin,
noradrenaline and enkephalins as transmitters. Further
processing of the pain stimuli goes rostrad through the
lateral spino-thalamic tract to the thalamus, but other
ascending pathways may also be involved[6]. The relative role
of the various nociceptive stimuli (pressure, vibration,
chemical, thermal, intense mechanical) in releasing the
stress-response remains to be determined as well as a

definite description of the peripheral substrates (transmitters) involved[5, 6, 7]. Thus we still have an imperfect
knowledge of the effect of various pain stimuli to release
the stress-response, and the role of pain in amplifying the
stress-response during and after surgery has therefore been
studied indirectly by looking at the influence of pain
alleviation on the endocrine-metabolic response to surgery.

Pain relief by antagonising peripheral mediators of
pain.

Although clinical studies have shown that prostaglandin
synthetase (cyclo-oxygenase) inhibitors may provide relief
of postoperative pain, no information is available on the
possible subsequent reduction in endocrine-metabolic
function, as well as no data have been published on the
influence of the administration of antihistamines, serotonin
antagonists and substance-P antagonists on the stress-
response.

Blockade of afferent pain transmission by regional
anaesthesia.

Several studies have demonstrated that most of the
classical endocrine-metabolic changes during and after
surgery may be blocked by both spinal and epidural analgesia
(review see 8). The influence of spinal anaesthesia is
transient and abates corresponding to the regression of the
sensory level of analgesia. A continuous epidural analgesia
is the most effective method to inhibit the stress-response
and this applies especially to procedures in the lower part
of abdomen (gynecological procedures) and procedures on the
lower extremities. In contrast, epidural analgesia has a
less modifying effect on the stress-response during major
(upper) abdominal procedures[8], probably because of the inability to establish a complete afferent blockade by
epidural analgesia. The open vagal afferent pathway may be
of minor importance in this context. Several studies have
demonstrated that postoperative pain relief by epidural
analgesia may not necessarily lead to a reduction in the
stress-response[8] probably because other afferent neurogenic

stimuli than pain stimuli may release the stress-response.
Thus, pain relief following hysterectomy may be achieved by
epidural analgesia with local anaesthetics with a level of
sensory analgesia extending from S_5 to T_8 or from S_5 to T_4.
However, a pronounced reduction of the cortisol and hyperglycemic response was only obtained during the extensive
blockade ($S_5 - T_4$) despite sufficient pain relief in both
groups[9]. This discrepancy between endocrine response and
pain relief during epidural analgesia has also been observed
by others[10]. Postoperative pain relief by splanchnic
blockade with lidocaine led to a reduction, but not
normalization, of oxygen uptake after cholecystectomy[11]. In
addition, there was no correlation between postoperative
pain relief by epidural analgesia and the stress-response as
assessed by urinary excretion of cortisol, catecholamines
and nitrogen neither when using a combination of local
anaesthetics and morphine[12] nor a regimen consisting of high
doses of bupivacaine (500-700 mg/day)[13]. These findings
again emphasize that pain stimuli are not the only release
mechanism of the stress-response to surgery.

Pain relief by modification of transmission of pain
stimuli in the dorsal horn.

Several studies have demonstrated that intrathecal or
epidural administration of opiates may lead to postoperative
pain relief and that this effect probably is mediated
through opiate receptors in the dorsal horn. However,
postoperative pain alleviation by epidural administration of
morphine following abdominal hysterectomy did only result in
a minor reduction of the hyperglycemic and cortisol response
[14, 15, 16]. Similar findings have been made during
cholecystectomy[17] and other abdominal procedures[12] with a
satisfactory pain treatment by epidural morphine administration but only a minor reduction in the stress-response, once
more emphasizing that pain stimuli is only one of several
release mechanisms of the stress-response.

Several clinical studies have shown that transcutaneous

electrical stimulation may provide some pain relief during
the postoperative period, and that this effect probably is
mediated through modulation of transmission of pain stimuli
in the dorsal horn, but no data have been published on the
influence on endocrine-metabolic changes. Similarly, no data
are available on the influence of administration of
substance-P antagonists or GABA mimetic drugs which also may
modify pain transmission at the dorsal horn level.

   Influence of pain relief by stimulation of inhibitory
descending pathways.

   No data from clinical studies.

   Influence of pain relief by systemic administration of
opiates.

   Although this technique has been extensively used for
postoperative pain relief limited data have been published
on the possible modifying effect on the endocrine-metabolic
response to surgery. Buprenorphine administration either im.
or i.v. had a slight and transient inhibitory effect on
postoperative changes in blood glucose and plasma cortisol[18].
In a preliminary study i.v. morphine (0.15 mg/kg/ led to a
pronounced reduction in plasma noradrenaline concomitant to
relief of pain, but without any significant inhibition of
the raised plasma cortisol levels[19]. Systemic administration
of opiates has also been described to reduce the postoperative increase in oxygen consumption, although not to
resting normal levels[11, 20].

   In summary, despite the many available techniques for
postoperative pain relief, we have a rather imperfect
knowledge on the influence of pain alleviation on the
endocrine-metabolic changes following surgical procedures
except for the modifying effect of regional anaesthesia.
Nevertheless, at this stage the following conclusions may be
made 1) stimuli leading to postoperative pain represent only
one of several release mechanisms of the stress-response to
surgery 2) pain relief per se by systemic or epidural

administration of opiates only partly reduces the stress-
response 3) pain relief by epidural administration of local
anaesthetics is more effective than opiates in reducing the
stress-response, despite a similar degree of pain relief 4)
no data exist on the influence of postoperative pain relief
by other pharmacological or physical means on the stress-
response.

With regard to the possible effect of pain relief on
postoperative morbidity the data from studies during regional anaesthesia suggest that some aspects of morbidity may
be mitigated following procedures in the lower part of the
body (prostatectomy and hip surgery)[21] while pain relief by
epidural analgesia may be less effective on morbidity
following abdominal (upper) procedures[22]. The influence of
postoperative pain relief by other pharmacological or
physical means on postoperative morbidity is presently unknown.

REFERENCES

1. Kehlet H. 1984. The stress-response to anaesthesia and
   surgery - release mechanisms and modifying factors.
   Clinics in Anaesthesiology 2: (in press).
2. Kehlet H. 1984. Pain relief and modification of the
   stress-response. In "Pain Management" Ed. G.D. Phillips
   and M.J. Cousins. Clinics in Critical Care Medicine.
   Churchill Livingston, London (in press).
3. Masek J & Horky J. 1957. Changes in nitrogen balance
   during chronic pain. Rev Czech Med 3: 42.
4. Güllner H-G, Nicholson WE, Wilson MG, Bartter C & Orth DN.
   1982. The response of plasma immunoreactive adrenocorti-
   cotropin, beta-endorphin/beta-lipotropin, ɣ -lipotropin
   and cortisol to experimentally induced pain in normal
   subjects. Clin Sci 63: 397.
5. Jessell TM. 1982. Neurotransmitters and CNS disease: Pain.
   Lancet ii: 1084.
6. Yaksh TL & Hammond DL. 1982. Peripheral and central
   substrates involved in the rostrad transmission of nociceptive information. Pain 13: 1.
7. Dubner R & Bennett GJ. 1983. Spinal and trigeminal
   mechanisms of nociception. Ann Rev Neurosci 6: 381.
8. Kehlet H. 1982. The modifying effect of general and
   regional anesthesia on the endocrine-metabolic response
   to surgery. Reg Anesth 7: S38.

9. Engquist A, Brandt MR, Fernandes A & Kehlet H. 1977. The blocking effect of epidural analgesia on the adrenocortical and hyperglycemic response to surgery. Acta Anaesth Scand 21: 330.

10. Lush D, Thorpe JN, Ricardson DJ, Bowen DJ. 1972. The effect of epidural analgesia on the adrenocortical response to surgery. Br J Anaesth 44: 1169.

11. Wiklund L. 1975. Splanchnic oxygen uptake during postoperative splanchnic blockade and postoperative fentanyl analgesia. Acta Anaesth Scand 19: 29.

12. Hjortsø N-C, Christensen NJ, Andersen T & Kehlet H. 1983. Influence of pain alleviation by epidural local anesthetics and morphine on urinary excretion of cortisol, catecholamines and nitrogen after abdominal surgery. Ann Surg (submitted).

13. Hjortsø N-C, Bigler D, Christensen NJ & Kehlet H. 1984. Influence of epidural analgesia with large doses of bupivacaine on the urinary excretion of cortisol, catecholamines and nitrogen after abdominal surgery. (in preparation).

14. Christensen P, Brandt MR, Rem J & Kehlet H. 1982. Influence of extradural morphine on the adrenocortical and hyperglycaemic response to surgery. Br J Anaesth 54: 24.

15. Jørgensen BC, Andersen HB & Engquist A. 1982. Influence of epidural morphine on postoperative pain, endocrine-metabolic, and renal responses to surgery: a controlled study. Acta Anaesthesiol Scand 26: 63.

16. Cowen MJ, Bullingham RES, Paterson GMC, McQuay HJ, Turner M, Allen MC. 1982. A controlled comparison of the effects of extradural diamorphine and bupivacaine on plasma glucose and plasma cortisol in postoperative patients. Anesth Analg 61: 15.

17. Rutberg H, Håkonsson E, Anderberg B, Jorfeldt L, Mårtensson J & Schildt B. 1984. Effects of extradural morphine and local anaesthetics on the endocrine response to upper abdominal surgery. Br J Anaesth (in press).

18. McQuay HJ, Bullingham RES, Paterson GMC & Moore RA. 1980. Clinical effects of buprenorphine during and after operation. Br J Anaesth 52: 1013.

19. Kothary SP & Zsigmond EK. 1980. Plasma cortisol and norepinephrine after pain relief. Int Congr Ser No. 537. Excerpta Medica, Amsterdam, p. 452.

20. Fournell A, Wilhelmy B, Falke K, Sandmann W & Böhmer G. 1980. Kontinuierliche Messung der Sauerstoffaufnahme bei postoperativer Periduralanalgesie. In "Neue Aspekte in der Regionalanaesthesie 1" Eds. HJ Wüst & M Zindler. Springer Verlag, Berlin, p. 54.

21. Kehlet H. 1983. Influence of regional anaesthesia on postoperative morbidity. In "Die kontinuierliche Periduralanaesthesie. Eds. J Meyer & H Nolte. Georg Thieme Verlag, Stuttgart, p. 75.

22. Hjortsø NC, Neumann P, Frøsig F, Andersen T, Lindhard A, Rogon E & Kehlet H. 1984. A controlled study on the effect of epidural analgesia with local anaesthetics and morphine on morbidity after abdominal surgery. (in preparation).

248